MW01280191

Macro Hacks

For more information about this title or to order other books and/or electronic media, contact the publisher:

Redefining Strength LLC
25651 Taladro Circle Suite G
Mission Viejo, CA
92691

(949) 287-3123

programs@redefiningstrength.com

www.redefiningstrength.com

ISBN: 978-0-578-88327-4

First Published 2019

Printed in PRC

Disclaimer & Copyright

The information provided in this book is designed to provide helpful information on the subjects discussed. This book is not meant to be used, nor should it be used, to diagnose or treat any medical condition. For diagnosis or treatment of any medical problem, consult your own physician. The publisher and author are not responsible for any specific health or allergy needs that may require medical supervision and aren't liable for any damages or negative consequences from any treatment, action, application, or preparation, to any person reading or following the information in this book. References are provided for informational purposes only and do not constitute endorsement of any websites or other sources.

This publication is protected under the US Copyright Act of 1976 and all other applicable international, federal, state and local laws, and all rights are reserved, including resale rights: you are not allowed to give or sell this Guide to anyone else. If you received this publication from anyone other than Redefining Strength you've received a pirated copy. Please contact us via email support at cori@redefiningstrength.com and notify us of the situation.

Although the author and publisher have made every reasonable attempt to achieve complete accuracy of the content in this Guide, they assume no responsibility for errors or omissions. Also, you should use this information as you see fit, and at your own risk. Your particular situation may not be exactly suited to the examples illustrated here; in fact, it's likely that they won't be the same, and you should adjust your use of the information and recommendations accordingly.

Any trademarks, service marks, product names or name features are assumed to be the property of their respective owners, and are used only for reference. There is no implied endorsement if we use one of these terms.

Finally, use your head. Nothing in this guide is intended to replace common sense, legal, medical or other professional advice, and is meant to inform the reader. So have fun with Redefining Strength, and get your stuff done.

Copyright © 2021 Redefining Strength LLC. All rights reserved worldwide.

Table of Contents

I'll give it to you straight…

The best diet for **YOU**?

It's the one you can **STICK TO**!

High protein. Low carb. Low fat…none of it really matters in the end if you can't create something that fits your lifestyle.

But even once you find a diet you can stick to, this doesn't mean you'll do one thing for the rest of your life!

For some reason, we've come to believe that we're going to find this MAGICAL diet we just want to do every single day and never stray from.

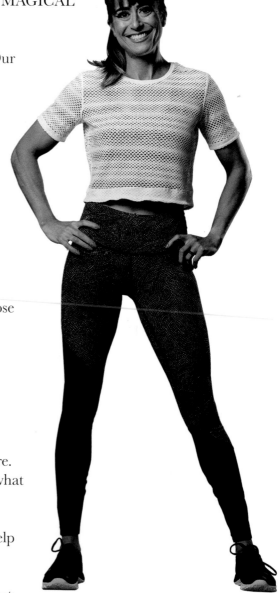

But our goals change. Our lifestyle changes. Our workouts adapt. Our schedules adjust…

Basically everything else in our life adapts and progresses over time.

So why wouldn't your diet, over time, adjust too?

There is no one size fits all plan. And no magical "lifestyle" you're going to do forever.

Your diet CAN and SHOULD adjust over time as your body and goals change.

The key is to understand the fundamentals of nutrition and how those building blocks of a healthy diet can be adjusted to meet your ever changing needs and goals.

Because one size doesn't fit all!

And that's why I've created this Macro Hacks guide.

I understand that there is a TON of conflicting information out there. It can be hard to figure out what is just a fad and a "quick fix" and what can truly help you get the results you're looking for.

And that's why I wanted to boil everything down to the basics - to help you "hack" that dieting code.

With these macro "hacks," I want to TEACH you how to eat well, but also I give you sample meal plans and recipes mapped out so you can have an easy place to start.

The Macro Hacks program is not another 6 week challenge or weight loss plan. It's not a quick fix...so if you're looking for that, you're in the wrong place.

It's a guide to help you dial in your nutrition based on YOUR needs and YOUR goals so you can achieve SUSTAINABLE results and have a healthy foundation off of which to build.

In the Macro Hacks guide, I'll help you understand the basics of nutrition - the building blocks of a healthy diet - and then show you how to tweak them to meet your needs and goals as they change over time.

Whether you're just starting out on your weight loss journey, looking to get a six pack, wanting to gain muscle, training for a marathon or simply dealing with those dreaded hormonal changes, I'll show you how you can adjust your diet to get results.

And I'll give you some delicious meals to enjoy on your way to achieving and MAINTAINING the lean, strong HEALTHY body you've always wanted!

So if you're ready to dial in your diet according to your specific needs and goals, my Macro Hacks are here to help!

Getting Started - Mindset Matters!?

Before you read any further...before you even start to make a change, I need you first to consider your MINDSET.

Yup...that's right...A proper MINDSET is key!

It sounds strange when talking about nutrition and healthy eating to first discuss mindset.

But if we don't have the right ATTITUDE toward making changes, no matter how much we may want a different result, we aren't going to make progress.

Too often our attitude holds us back, causing us to fail before we even really get started.

It is key you realize that CHANGE IS HARD.

Tracking, learning a new way of eating...heck sometimes even staying dedicated to your goals when life tries to get in the way is hard!

Change always is!

But if you want a new and better result, you've got to be willing to risk "failing" - you've got to be prepared to make the hard change.

If you commit though 100% to a new plan and really go ALL IN, you WILL see progress. You just need to remember that the process can seem scary and intimidating to start.

While I will provide tips to help make everything easier, I do think it is key you recognize that it can be difficult to make changes no matter how small.

Giving yourself CREDIT for taking the risk too, can make everything else easier even.

Just remember there will be a learning curve!

Reach out any time you need help or a boost. You have access to an amazing private group with people at all stages in their fitness journey ready to help you out and support you!

And here are 4 tips that will help you ease your fears and get in the right mindset to succeed!

4 Tips To Make CHANGE Easier

If you don't trust the process, your plan is doomed before you even get started.

But part of what holds us back from jumping in head first is that fear of failure.

We don't want to make these massive changes only to have things not work out.

And it's kind of funny we have this fear because often we are looking to make a change in the first place because the things we're currently doing aren't working as well as we'd like.

But despite the fact that our current plan isn't working, it's at least familiar. And that makes it "safe."

Another thing that often happens is, when we are faced with having to make a change, we often try to JUSTIFY or DEFEND what we've been doing.

But we have to get it out of our heads that making a change means we were "wrong" to start.

Because your diet may not have been "wrong" or unhealthy.

Yup...you can be doing a whole bunch of "good" things and still not be getting the results you want, especially if your goals have changed!

It's why sometimes small tweaks can make the difference.

And you may find these Macro Hacks simply help you make those final "tweaks" to get the results you want.

So don't feel like you just have to throw away everything you were doing.

Just remember, no matter how "healthy" or even well-researched our plan is, over time we may have to tweak it.

Your goals and needs CHANGE and the key is understanding how we can react to these changes over time to keep progressing and getting the results we want!

Before you jump right in and even get overwhelmed by the options, I wanted to share 4 tips I tell my clients, especially if they're feeling a bit nervous or resistant to the change.

These 4 tips are:

1 **Start today!**

2 **Set habit goals**

3 **Stop the guilt**

4 **Set boundaries - but stop labeling things as bad and good**

So while, especially #4, may seem obvious..."knowing" these tips and actually IMPLEMENTING them are two different things.

Let's start by breaking things down so you can take some action TODAY.

If you're reading this right now, you're motivated to make a change. And you want to take advantage of this motivation and dive right in!

1. No Matter What - Start today!

Our initial motivation fades quickly. The key is using it to our advantage when we can.

It would be really easy to read this book today, put it down figuring you'll start tomorrow/Monday/on the first... and never actually take that first step.

The best way to take advantage of the motivation that lead you to start reading this is to do SOMETHING as soon as you can.

Because knowing we've started, even if it is something small, can help us continue to stay motivated.

I think often the reason many of us don't start immediately is because we claim we are "all or nothing" people.

We think that if we can't do everything at once and do the plan perfectly, we just can't start.

And there is nothing wrong with taking a day to read everything and jumping in head first, making all the changes at once.

I get it...some of us like to cannonball into a cold pool and get the shock all at once instead of slowly submerging inch by inch, letting each body part adapt before we continue.

But if the idea of making all of the changes at once feels overwhelming, or if you're using this as an EXCUSE to wait for some magical "perfect time"...well...it would be much better to pick one change to make today.

Don't let this all or nothing attitude become an EXCUSE to not really begin something...trust me I've personally used this one far too many times.

Because really the question you have to ask yourself is "Why?"

Why do you really need to wait till you can do it all at once? Why wouldn't at least doing one thing TODAY help you make progress?

Let's face it...it would.

Even if you have a plan to go "all in" on Monday, why not do one thing today?

One change MAY get you moving forward even before you can implement the others.

And one change at a time is MANAGEABLE.

I also think realizing that one little change can make a difference can really help us create a lifestyle.

There are going to be times where you slightly go off plan. Life is going to "get in the way."

You aren't always going to be perfectly motivated.

And having the attitude of "all or nothing" only lends itself to you completely giving up and feeling like you've "ruined a day" if you do one thing off track.

Part of truly creating a lifestyle is realizing there will be times you more strictly adhere to your plan to reach specific goals and other times you are a bit more relaxed with it and just enjoy.

It means also realizing that one little change can make all the difference.

So as you start to dive into all of this information, think about one change you can make TODAY.

Even if you simply make out a grocery list to prep for tomorrow or start outlining a plan.

Do one thing you can check off your list and confidently tell yourself was a start!

Do one thing you can build on tomorrow!

2. Set Habit Goals

You probably didn't start reading this guide because you had specific habits you wanted to accomplish.

No...we most often want to make diet changes to lose weight/gain muscle/get a six pack/improve our health or some combination of these things.

But on our way to accomplishing these goals, we need to create new habits to support them.

That's why it's key we actually set specific HABIT GOALS.

Progress is NEVER linear. There will be ups and downs.

Days you gain weight on the scale even though you stuck to the plan perfectly (a subject I'll be going into later).

And because there will be ups and downs along the way, you've got to have a way to make yourself trust the process if you want long term success.

The best way to do that and convince yourself you're heading in the right direction, even when sometimes it doesn't feel that way, is to track your habit changes and make those changes part of your goals!

If you make a commitment to enacting certain habits each week, aka you make those habit changes a GOAL, you can ensure you'll get the other results you ultimately want.

You can also keep yourself motivated along the way by REWARDING yourself for achieving those habit changes - changes you are more in control of on a day to day basis.

Too often we wait to reward ourselves until we reach our ultimate goal" change when to until. The bigger your goal, the longer you'll have to wait to recognize your progress.

The bigger the goal, the more long-term it is, the easier it is to get discouraged as you ignore the little changes occurring because you still aren't "there yet".

That's why you want to set habit goals, track them and REWARD yourself for achieving them. Because those goals are the building blocks of your success.

So as you read through and write down the changes you want to implement, break them down into daily and weekly habits.

Make those habits a goal and set a way to reward yourself for making those changes!

3. Stop The Guilt

But what if you DON'T stick to the new habits one day?

What if you "slip up?"

Did you ruin the day?

NOPE!

And that is one of the most important things we have to remember when making changes.

Often it isn't the actual thing we did that derails our progress. It's the fact that we make ourselves feel GUILTY for doing it.

That guilt is what leads to use eating other things we didn't plan and into what many call that yo-yo dieting cycle.

What does this cycle look like?

You eat according to your goals but then life/stress/family gets in the way. You have one little thing "off plan."

You then feel guilty and feel like you've ruined the day. So you eat more.

Who cares, right? It's already ruined.

But what could have been one little thing, ends up turning into not only a whole day, but even 2 or 3 days.

It snowballs until you end up feeling like you're starting all over again.

It doesn't have to be that way though.

And the way to prevent that from happening isn't by expecting ourselves to be perfect - it's by stopping the guilt!

So as you start to implement new habits, don't expect yourself to be perfect with them.

Even PLAN for that first "slip up."

By plan I mean recognize that it will happen and that the best thing you can do is take it in stride, ENJOY IT, and move forward.

Think about things this way...If you got a flat tire on your car, would you then slash the other three?

No, you'd do what you can to fix it and move forward!

Same goes for your diet.

If you eat a cookie, or even two or three or 7, don't just decide your day is ruined and say "F%^$ it" then get pizza and ice cream too. NOPE!

Just move forward.

Maybe it does mean making it your cheat day and steering into the skid if you decide to include cheat days.

Maybe that is easiest so you don't feel guilty.

Or maybe it means not hitting your macros but having the healthy meal you planned after just to keep moving forward.

The key is you want to enjoy those indulgences instead of feeling guilty about them because the guilt is what leads to you causing damage that doesn't need to be done!

Just remember that first indulgence may be a flat tire, but you don't want to do your own car in by going and slashing the other three tires!

4. Set Boundaries - But Stop Labeling Things As Bad And Good!

Most of us need boundaries to succeed. They give us direction and hold us accountable.

And the more clearly we outline these guidelines for ourselves, often the better our results.

BUT we need to recognize that setting boundaries is something completely different than labeling foods as "good" and "bad" or "off limits" and "clean."

While it may seem silly that I'm talking about the terms we use to create our guidelines, these terms relate back to our mindset. They can influence how much GUILT we feel if we deviate from our plan.

When you label foods as "unclean" or "bad," it makes sense you'd feel bad or guilty if you ate them.

If you want to set boundaries around the types of foods you eat, because, yes, you want more nutrient-dense foods to make up the bulk of your diet for your health and better results faster, consider instead making a list of foundational foods

Create a list of foods you want to make the foundation of your diet and then try to primarily pick from this food list.

You're giving yourself direction and boundaries without saying a food not on that list is bad.

You're pushing yourself toward foods that may be more beneficial for your health while still allowing yourself to eat other things and ENJOY the foods you love.

Same goes for making things "off limits."

Ever notice how the second you tell yourself you can't have something, you want it all the more?

Not to mention, you feel WAY more guilty if you eat something that is completely off limits.

Again focus on the foods you want to be eating. Put the emphasis on what you want to be consuming over what you shouldn't be eating.

And even give yourself guidelines that don't demand perfection when it comes to your food choices.

The 80/20 rule is an amazing way to think about food quality. 80% of the time, you want your calories to come from those foods you know are nutrient-dense. They are whole, natural foods you know your body and health benefit from.

While the other 20% of your calories CAN come from foods you enjoy, but well...you know aren't necessarily the best for you.

By knowing you can see results while still indulging, you give yourself direction and guidelines to steer you in the right direction without any of the guilt or the extreme restriction we can feel with some diets when given a "clean foods" list.

The key is giving yourself guidelines that aren't so repressive. Because the more we restrict, often the more likely we are at some point to rebel and go back to the habits we'd like to change!

Now...TRACK To Keep Yourself On Track!

Once you set habit goals and create guidelines, you need to make sure to track what you are doing and how things are going.

It's really easy to overlook small changes as they add up or even ignore the times we take "liberties" with our plan.

The more we track, the better the results we can get because we can see what is and isn't working to tweak our plan as we go.

Tracking also creates accountability. It shows us what we need to do and gives us that little nudge to do the habits we know we should even on those days we don't want to!

So as you go through making changes, make sure you've written down your goals, you've set ways to measure even small progress toward them and you set a consistent time to measure - whether it is weighing daily to average your progress or measuring once a week or every couple of weeks.

You also need to track your actual IMPLEMENTATION of your plan.

Too often we "feel" like we are doing all of the right things when, in reality, we aren't actually fully sticking to our plan. And if we can look back and see what we've done exactly, we can also understand why things are, or maybe aren't, working.

So when you're making diet changes, as much as you may hate it, you've got to log your food, especially when you first start out!

Why You Need To Log And Track Your Food...

It's not exactly fun to measure and enter the meals or recipes or ingredients.

It's annoying to look everything up. To weigh and measure every little thing you eat. (To even sort through the incorrect foods in many trackers).

It can be annoying to take the time to enter everything or even tweak our meals to hit specific macro breakdowns.

But if you want to make sure something will work...If you want to GUARANTEE yourself results, you NEED to track.

We often don't realize the true macronutrient breakdown of the foods we eat. Or the calories that certain foods contain.

Plus...portions are easily distorted.

Simply not eating everything on your plate at a restaurant may still mean you're eating more calories than you realize.

Even when we eyeball our portion sizes at home, it can be hard to tell exactly what we're getting.

Those portions would look basically the EXACT SAME to us eyeballing them.

Can You Spot The Difference?

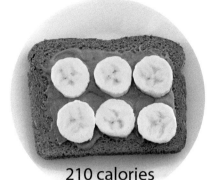
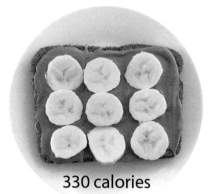

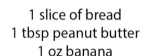

210 calories

330 calories

1 slice of bread
1 tbsp peanut butter
1 oz banana

1 slice of bread
2 tbsp peanut butter
2.4 oz banana

Crap they look the same to me even now.

There are so many things that can factor into what we "feel" is a proper portion if we haven't measured…like even simply how much we WANT, or don't want, to eat something.

And it is easy for those little snacks we eat throughout the day, that almost go unnoticed, to add up.

That "bite" you took of something can add up more quickly than you realize.

Because it isn't just those few extra calories one day, but the fact that we are often doing them day in and day out over the entire course of a week, a month…a year.

That's why we need the accountability of logging as it paints an accurate picture of what we are truly doing - the macronutrients we are giving our body, the quality of the foods we are eating and also the calorie intake we're consuming.

It is a teaching tool to help us see how different foods affect us so we can learn true hunger signals and what proper portions look like. For a chart to help you recognize portion sizes using your hand, see page 188.

It is the way we can get back to eating more "intuitively."

We can re-learn how to really respond to what our bodies need as often a lack of sleep, stress, boredom or simple enjoying the taste can distort those intuitive signals.

If we don't track, we don't really 100% know what we are doing. It's why we can "feel" like we are doing all of the right things yet not getting the results we want…

Think of the frustration we feel as diet after diet fails because…well…we don't SEE those extras adding up.

If we've tracked, we can easily go back and make small tweaks. Or even clearly see where we've fallen off.

But without tracking, we just don't know!

Is that frustration, consistent yo-yoing and failure really better than a few minutes spent tracking daily?

I don't think so!

Especially because tracking becomes easier and easier the more you do it and save your meals to use later.

It really comes down to pick your sucky...

Be unhappy that you aren't seeing the results you want when you are 100% working hard or be slightly annoyed you have to weigh and measure and track, especially at the start.

I can tell you which I'd prefer...And one becomes habit so in the end it doesn't really take any time at all or even register as a task...

No matter what diet hybrid you create, and especially if you want to build a LIFESTYLE, you need to first understand what truly works and how it affects you!

So if you're committed to truly making a change and creating a new lifestyle, you've got to LEARN how to eat accordingly and that means tracking to start!

Now...Do I Have To Track Forever?

The simple answer? No!

Tracking is to help you understand what you are truly consuming and to guide you when you're working toward a specific goal.

Especially if you aren't familiar with macronutrients and the proportions of protein, carbs and fat, tracking is essential. And often eye opening!

But once you understand how to properly fuel, you may decide you don't need to track anymore, especially if you're just continuing to MAINTAIN your results.

We can learn to listen to our body and accept a bit more deviation in our portions and macros when we're just working to maintain our current situation.

However, if you set a specific goal to achieve, tracking becomes essential. ESPECIALLY if this is your first time making a specific change or working toward a specific goal.

You may decide you want to gain "x" amount of muscle.

So you track.

You may decide you want to lose a little bit of extra fat for your big birthday.

So you track.

Basically, understanding how to track gives you the ability to more efficiently reach your goals and even understand HOW you actually got there.

Too often when we don't log and make a ton of changes, we don't know what actually worked. This can make it incredibly difficult for us to achieve those same, or better, results later on!

So think of logging and tracking like studying for a test.

It's the best way to "guarantee" you get the grade you want while also helping you understand the information to use later on!

3 Tips To Help You Use A Food Tracker

So the idea of logging everything...well let's face it, it's not really something any of us "want" to do.

But there are some things you can do before you even really start tracking daily to set yourself up for success.

These 3 tips will make your day to day tracking easier because you've done the prep work!

-Save recipes, meals and ingredients.
-Log "sample" days.
-Get a scale.

1. Save Recipes, Meals and Ingredients

Instead of having to search for the ingredients every time, most food trackers, like My Fitness Pal, allow you to save recipes or meals.

This way you can have your own library of meals to enter without having to search each and every time for the ingredients.

Also, if you make a recipe you've found online that lists the macros for a serving, create a "food" with the name of the recipe and list the macros they've given you. As long as you don't make swaps but use the same basic ingredients (even if slightly different brands), your macro and calorie breakdown will be within a few grams which is precise enough.

You then don't have to search for each ingredient again, which saves time. Plus, the next time you want to make that recipe, or even eat the leftovers the next day, you can easily just "add" the food to your log!

Basically, the more you create your own database of meals and recipes you use frequently before you start logging, the easier the day to day tracking will be!

You can even share recipes between friends and family members by texting them a link!

It's also important to know...there is natural deviation in the foods we eat. Two apples, even ones that weigh the same, may have slightly different amounts of calories and sugars.

However, very little deviations shouldn't be stressed over.

BUT you do want to note there will be massive deviations sometimes in the foods/ingredients logged in those food trackers.

And some aren't correct.

I've seen a piece of chocolate cake listed with 1,000 calories and one with 10....

It can be good to double check ingredients to find the most "accurate" or agreed upon calorie and macro breakdown.

This way you can be as exact as possible and as consistent as possible in your logs!

2. Log Sample Days

You've selected your goal and found your starting plan and you're excited to get started. What can you do today?

I recommend logging "sample" days for yourself.

These days help you plan ahead and see where tweaks need to be made to your diet. They also show you the macro breakdowns of the foods you eat.

Plus, they allow you to still enjoy the foods you want while creating a meal plan for yourself.

Even if you log some of the days in this plan and use those recipes, you then have all of that saved to easily add at other times.

And when you have this base already planned out, if your plans change during the day or week, you can simply adjust the foundation.

Especially to start, this is far easier than planning days as you go!

I even find planning two "sample" days of meals for yourself can allow you to meal prep for half the week on Sunday and then the other half on Wednesday. This keeps things simple, but also gives you a bit of variety so you aren't just eating the exact same thing 6-7 days a week!

3. Get A Scale

While there is going to be deviation in the exact foods we eat, and precision is really a slightly relative term when counting calories and macros, the more you can have a CONSISTENT measurement yourself, the better off you'll be.

Basically, if you measure in the same way, you'll at least have consistency across your readings.

And the most accurate way to measure is using a food scale.

From weighing out the raw ingredients, to even dividing recipes, this is the best way to make sure you're consistently eating the same portions.

Now...you may be thinking, how can I make sure I get an accurate portion when I make a recipe that may have meat and veggies and potatoes all mixed together?

Don't stress over counting the exact number of chicken chunks in the portion you get!

We have to remember with all of this it isn't just the meal or the day that matters, but our consistency over the weeks and months.

When you have a recipe, weigh the entire dish then divide it out into equal weighing portions paying attention to the fact that you don't give all the potatoes on one day and all the meat on another.

But don't stress otherwise.

Realize there is an amount of standard deviation we just have to accept.

Just know you're getting the most accurate reading using the scale!

(And added bonus, you don't need to clean up measuring cups or tablespoons if you happen to be in the US and use those frequently now!)

Set yourself up for success with a food tracker and take the time to learn that BEFORE you make changes. Test weighing out your foods and log what you are currently doing.

Create your own little database of recipes, meals and foods! This way you can even have go-to meals out!

Now, What Are These Macros You Speak Of?

Just about every diet out there boils down to MACROS.

They may claim they don't, and tell you that you don't have to track your macros, but by eliminating foods, they are creating specific macronutrient breakdowns.

Even the standard American diet has a common macro breakdown of 20% protein, 50% carbs and 30% fat.

So...What are macros?

Macros or macronutrients are the nutrients we need in large quantities - the protein, carbs and fats that make up the foods we eat.

Manipulating how many of our calories come from each macro can drastically change the results we get and how we fuel our bodies. It's why, based on our goals and training regimes, we may even change ratios over time.

The amount of each macro we consume can even impact how many calories we really need and the calorie surplus or deficit we create.

So how many calories are in a gram of each macro?

1 gram of PROTEIN contains 4 calories

1 gram of CARBS contains 4 calories
1 gram of FAT contains 9 calories

Fat is more calorically dense, which is often why people will say fat is more satiating.

However, because fat is more calorically dense, it can also feel like you get to eat very little fat before those calories really add up. This can lead to people overeating foods such as nuts so that they are no longer in the calorie deficit they need to lose weight.

Now you may be thinking, you're talking about how every diet boils down to macros, but if I eat less than I burn, won't I lose weight no matter what?

Isn't losing weight or gaining muscles really simply about calories in vs. calories out?

And yes...Calories 100% matter.

If you eat more than you burn, you'll gain weight.

If you eat less than you burn, you will lose weight.

BUT too often we focus only on eating more or less and not on where those calories are coming from.

And honestly, this is why so many of us are constantly "on a diet" or searching for something new.

Because results aren't just about calories in vs. calories out, but about what TYPE of calories we are consuming.

If we take the time to focus on where those calories are coming from (the macros we are consuming), we can get better results faster and MAINTAIN those results long term.

Think about it this way...you wouldn't put regular gas into an expensive sports car, right!?

It wouldn't run well and may even break down. Same thing happens when you eat low quality foods and improper macro ratios.

Plus, by dailing in your macros you can feel fuller and more energized.

200 calories of chips won't make you feel as full as 200 calories of meat and veggies even though they are technically both 200 calories.

And even if you're in a calorie deficit while eating certain foods, you may find that you don't get the same results as when you simply adjust your macronutrient breakdown!

The thermic effect of not only quality foods, but specific macros, as well as the satiating effect of specific macros and the nutrient-density of specific foods, all play a part in how our calorie intake affect our results and even the deficit we actually need to get those results.

The type, and quality, of our calories DOES really matter not only for results, but also for long-term adherence.

It's not simply calories in vs. calories out if you want results!

Why It's NOT Just Calories In Vs Calories Out

I've heard people say "a calorie is just a calorie." It is a measure of energy.

And while that is to some extent true, one calorie equals one calorie when it goes into our body, how our body UTILIZES that calorie can dramatically impact, not only how many calories we actually need, BUT the results we get from our diet (whether we want to gain muscle, lose weight or even better fuel our sport).

1000lbs of feathers and 1000lbs of bricks weigh the same, right? They are both 1000lbs.

But you also know a feather is lighter than a brick!

You won't dispute these things are dramatically different...especially if one is thrown at your head.

The same holds true for calories. While a calorie may be a calorie, the TYPE of calorie can impact how full you feel, the results you get and even your health.

It's why it's key we pay attention to our macros. The amount of our calorie intake that comes from each macro can change how that calorie impacts our body.

Each macro has a different function in our body, which impacts how our body runs and can affect how full we feel and even the number of calories we burn while at "rest."

When you first start by focusing on macros to dial in your calorie intake, you can make sure you're giving your body truly what it needs!

But before you can pick a macro ratio based on your goals, you need to understand the benefit of each macronutrient!

The Function Of Each Macro - Why No Macronutrient Is Evil!

Let's make one thing clear...No macronutrient is inherently evil.

Yes, if you have specific diseases or health issues, you may need to eliminate specific foods or reduce your intake of a specific macro, but for most of us that are healthy and "normal"...well...we need to stop just DEMONIZING a macro for no reason.

Carbs don't make you fat. Neither does fat.

Too often macros become demonized because of the few that do have special needs. But just because your friend needs to restrict carbs doesn't mean YOU need to or even should!

We need to dial in each macro based on our needs, our goals, our training routine and even our metabolic flexibility.

But before we can select the ratios right for us, we need to understand more about the function of each macro in the body and how it can impact our results.

Let's Talk About Protein:

Often we are told about "healthy" carbs and "healthy" fats. We are told to eat our fruits and vegetables. But what about PROTEIN!?

Why does it seem that we aren't really told about the importance of protein, other than maybe if we stray into bodybuilding realms?

It's actually kind of crazy we aren't saying "get enough healthy protein" as often as we're saying "eat your fruits and vegetables" because protein is literally what we're made up of!

Protein is key if we want to improve our performance, lose fat, gain muscle and even stay healthy and active as we get older!

Because protein sources not only contain important MICROnutrients our body needs, but protein is the building blocks of our bodily tissues!

If we don't get enough protein, we will start to plunder it from other parts of our body, meaning we will even break down muscle tissue to release the protein we need to support other bodily functions!

And ladies...think you need less protein?

You're wrong! Protein is even more important for you, especially if you're going through menopause or are post-menopausal!

So What Is Protein?

Proteins are made up of amino acids joined together by chemical bonds. These amino acid chains are folded together in different ways to create 3-D structures that are essential to our body's functioning.

And there are two main types of amino acids - essential and nonessential.

Essential amino acids can't be manufactured by our body and therefore must be consumed.

Some "essential" amino acids are conditionally essential. This means that we can't always create as much as we need, like, for instance, if we are under a ton of stress.

The second type, nonessential, are the amino acids our body can create for itself.

We need amino acids readily available in our blood to help our body produce important molecules like enzymes, hormones, neurotransmitters and even antibodies.

We also need these amino acids, proteins, available in our body to help us promote protein synthesis so we can get the results we work so hard to create in the gym - aka building lean muscle!

And while we most often think of protein as MEAT or coming from animals, you CAN also get a complete amino acid chain by combining different vegetable sources. I'll go over complementary proteins later on and you can learn the best sources of plant-based protein in the Know Your Veggies chart on page 185.

Why Is Protein So Important?

We are literally made up of protein.

From our bones to our muscles to our arteries and veins...heck even our skin, hair, and fingernails are made up of protein not to mention our heart, brain, liver, kidneys, and lungs are built from tissues made up of proteins!

Consuming adequate amounts of protein is key to keeping our tissues healthy and helping them repair and rebuild.

Protein helps replace worn out cells, transport substances throughout the body and even aids in growth and repair.

And yes, protein is the building blocks of muscle. So if you want to gain lean muscle mass, consuming an adequate amount of protein is key.

But don't fear that protein will make you "bulky!"

Protein can't make you pack on pounds of muscle.

We often hear that you can't out exercise a bad diet, but you can't out diet a bad workout routine either.

While increasing protein can help you build lean muscle, this will ONLY happen if you pair a higher protein diet with a proper training routine.

So if gaining muscle is your goal, make sure your workouts match your diet!

Challenge your body so that it is forced to rebuild stronger. Then make sure that you're adequately supporting protein synthesis by giving your body the amino acids it needs to rebuild!

But protein isn't just important for gaining muscle.

Actually, increasing protein may be even MORE BENEFICIAL for those of us looking to lose weight and change our body composition, especially as we get older.

Not only can the thermic effect of protein make losing weight on a higher protein diet EASIER, but increasing your protein while in a calorie deficit can help you retain your lean muscle mass to keep your metabolism strong and "healthy."

And retaining lean muscle mass is so key during weight loss and body recomposition because it keeps our resting metabolic rate as high as possible!

Now...what if you could actually BUILD muscle even while in a deficit?

Heard it's not possible, right?

Many of us have been told you can't lose fat AND build muscle at the same time.

Well, that's not exactly true.

While it is a slower process, studies have shown that high protein diets can actually help you even BUILD lean muscle mass while in a DEFICIT.

So not only can increasing your protein intake directly help you lose weight, but it can indirectly help you lose weight by allowing you to increase lean muscle mass and keep your resting metabolic rate higher.

Plus, having more lean muscle mass and less fat means you'll look even leaner than if you'd simply lost weight on a scale!

How Can Increasing Protein Help You Lose Weight?

There are 3 main reasons that you need to focus on protein if your goal is to lose weight or change your body composition (aka lose fat).

These 3 main reasons high protein is key are:

1 **Protein has a high thermic effect**

2 **Protein is more satiating and promotes optimal functioning**

3 **Protein can help you maintain, and even gain, lean muscle to avoid metabolic adaptation during your calorie deficit**

1: Protein has a high thermic effect

So what the heck is the "thermic effect" of food?

The thermic effect, or thermogenic effect, of food is the calories you expend to digest and process the food.

Protein takes the most energy to digest with about 20-30% of the total calories in protein eaten going to digesting it. Then carbs take about 5-10% while fats take 0-3%.

Studies have even shown protein to have a thermogenic effect 5 times greater than carbs or fat!

Basically, you burn more calories to process protein than you do the other macros.

So when you're setting your caloric intake, you need to consider the amount of each macro you are consuming.

Because consuming a 1,500 calorie diet of more carbs and fat and a 1,700 calorie diet with higher protein may be the same deficit at the end of the day.

It's why a calorie isn't just a calorie and you need to consider your macros first.

If you choose a ratio higher in protein, you may find you need to increase your overall caloric intake even if your goal is to create a calorie deficit.

You can also use the thermic effect of protein to your advantage to avoid weight loss plateaus by adjusting protein ratios over your weight loss journey.

Often when our progress stalls, we think we need to cut our calories lower.

Not only can this hold us back, but it can be why we end up falling off our diet or struggling to maintain our results. It can also lead to more muscle mass loss, which can then negatively impact our metabolic rate and again hinder our progress.

We want to preserve our lean muscle mass as much as possible by getting enough protein otherwise we will catabolize our muscle mass in order to make protein available for our other bodily needs!

So if you've hit a plateau, try first adjusting protein levels.

And as you get closer to your goal, especially if you're shooting for lower levels of body fat to reveal that six pack, you may actually find the thermic effect benefits you more!

Instead of implementing some crazy calorie restriction to get lean, utilize the fact that your body is more sensitive to the thermic effects of food and dial in your protein!

2: Protein is more satiating and promotes optimal functioning

Being hungry sucks. It can make you angry and grumpy. Actually, this is such a common thing during diets that we've come up with a word for it…

HANGER.

And while changing up your diet so you can lose weight can mean feeling a bit hungry as you first adapt, it really shouldn't be this miserable thing where you're constantly starving.

It shouldn't be this constant battle to not eat.

To help yourself avoid the hanger, feel energized, and even actually satisfied with your meals, so you can stick to your plan and get lasting results, you'll want to make sure your meals all focus on protein.

Protein helps us feel fuller for longer.

It's actually a satiating superstar because it triggers the release of hormones in our gut that tell us we are full so we not only stop eating, but can actually end up getting "full" off of eating fewer calories.

While I mentioned before you may find you actually can consume MORE calories while still losing weight if your diet is higher in protein, you may also find that a diet rich in protein is so FILLING, you end up eating less!

Again, another reason why we need to first focus on those macros to then dial in our calorie intake.

Getting enough protein is also key to helping your body run efficiently.

When your body is functioning optimally, your weight loss results are going to be better.

They're going to be better simply because you'll be able to perform more quality workouts with improved recovery between sessions due to your high protein fueling.

And on top of helping you benefit more from your workouts, protein can increase levels of the hormone glucagon. This hormone helps control body fat by causing the liver to release stored energy into circulation.

It can also help to liberate free fatty acids from adipose (fat) tissue. These free fatty acids are another way to get fuel for cells and make our body fat do something useful instead of lazily being stored around our stomachs!

3: Protein can help you maintain, and even gain, lean muscle to avoid metabolic adaptation during your calorie deficit

Many of us have heard that we can "damage" our metabolism by cutting calories too low. We've heard our metabolism can "slow down" because of going on a diet.

And both are to some extent true.

When you lose weight and you have less body mass, you naturally need fewer calories for your body to run.

But how much your metabolism slows down, or ADAPTS, is also dependent on how you diet.

The more restrictive your calorie intake is, aka the more extreme your deficit is in an attempt to lose weight quickly, the more muscle mass you may catabolize.

Our body seeks out the energy and nutrients it needs to function and will break down muscle tissue if needed to get them. It doesn't necessarily only draw energy from our fat mass (although increasing our protein intake CAN help us not only protect our muscle mass, but promote energy being preferentially drawn from our fat stores!).

When we restrict our calories and create more extreme deficits, we often also end up causing ourselves to be less active throughout the day and our workouts suffer. Let's face it when you don't have enough fuel, you feel tired and want to lounge around!

So our metabolism ADAPTS to our current needs and slows down. We simply don't need as many calories to function.

This is why focusing on higher protein, especially during a calorie deficit, is so key!

While your metabolism WILL adapt as you lose weight, you can prevent it from dropping lower than necessary by retaining and even BUILDING lean muscle mass through a high protein diet (and of course a proper workout routine).

The more muscle you have, the more calories you burn at rest. It's why even though your goal may be weight loss, you truly want to focus on losing fat.

Fat mass doesn't require as much energy to be maintained as muscle mass does. It's why often we can feel like we've damaged our metabolism in our attempts to lose weight quickly.

So increasing our protein to protect our lean muscle mass and even help us GAIN muscle while in a calorie deficit can help us avoid metabolic adaptation and keep our metabolism going strong!

Higher Protein Is Even More Important As You Get Older?!

Protein is not just an important macronutrient to focus on when we have aesthetic goals - when we want to lose weight or gain muscle.

Actually, one of the most important reasons to increase your protein intake may be your AGE.

As we get older, especially for you ladies out there, it can be harder and harder to retain and even GAIN lean muscle mass.

This loss of muscle mass can not only negatively impact our ability to stay active and injury-free, but it can also have consequences for our metabolic health.

It can feel like it gets harder and harder to not only lose weight, but even maintain the weight you've been at for years as you get older.

And part of this is because our metabolism naturally does slow down, but also because we aren't burning as many calories at rest due to a reduction in lean muscle mass.

But the answer isn't cutting calories lower, which may actually only backfire, causing you to catabolize MORE muscle tissue.

Instead, you need to focus on increasing your protein intake!

Yup...as you get older, your protein requirements may actually increase.

Consuming more protein as you get older is important because you simply don't process protein as efficiently as you once did.

And getting enough protein will not only be key to fighting against the loss of lean muscle mass so you can stay active and injury-free, but to improving your overall quality of life (and of course keeping you looking amazing at the same time!).

As we get older a diet higher in protein isn't just important for muscle retention.

Getting enough protein can also help us keep our immune system strong and prevent increased skin fragility.

And ladies between the ages of 55 and 92, do you want to improve your bone density and lessen your risk for osteoporosis? Then you need to increase your protein intake!

Studies showed that women between 55 to 92 who ate more protein had a higher bone density!

So especially if you are over 65, make sure you're focusing on that protein intake!

But, What If I'm Not Working Out Currently - Is Protein Still Key?

The short answer? Yes!

Protein is still key even if you aren't working out.

While consuming a high protein diet without resistance training won't help you gain muscle, a high protein diet can still help you protect your lean muscle mass and even lose weight.

And if you aren't training because of an injury?

Well then focusing on protein is actually even more important!

When we are injured, we often think we need less protein because we aren't training hard, but a diet higher in protein can help us prevent muscle loss as we rest while also improving our recovery.

Protein is the building blocks of muscle as well as our connective tissues and tendons.

An injury to those tissues means our body needs to repair, and since tendons and connective tissues tend to take longer to recover, it's even more important we do everything to provide them with the fuel they need aka MORE PROTEIN!

Greater protein synthesis accelerates tissue repair and strengthens connective tissues to reduce your future risk for injury as well.

And not only can a higher protein diet help you recover from injury, but it can also help you avoid gaining weight while your activity is reduced.

Because of thermogenic effect of protein, eating a higher protein diet can help you prevent excess fat gain even when you're in an "overfed" state.

You don't want to cut calories too low when you're out with an injury because you want to help your body recover; however, you also don't want to gain a ton of fat while you're not as active.

Keeping your protein high can help you avoid gaining a ton of fat even when you aren't training!

What Really Constitutes High Protein?

That is a question up for debate....

The standard American diet, the ratio you'll see in most fitness trackers, puts protein at 20%. Daily recommendations for the minimum amount needed put us at about 10%.

At about 10% we are getting about .8 grams of protein per kilogram of bodyweight or about .36 grams per pound.

The problem with this minimum recommended number is that this number is really the amount we need to prevent protein DEFICIENCY.

It's not about getting an OPTIMAL amount, especially for those training hard.

So while you may "survive" we aren't just seeking survival...We actually want our bodies to THRIVE.
This puts active people seeking more in the range of 25-40% protein if they want to benefit from their training routine.

Many high protein diets will recommend between 30-50% of your diet come from protein and around that 30% is where you'll really start to see the benefits of a "high protein" diet.

The International Society of Sports Nutrition even recommends between 1.4-2 grams per pound for active people stating that it isn't only safe, but may actually improve training adaptations.

While there may not be "more" benefit to eating above 40% in terms of increased growth or weight loss for the average exerciser, many people will find success with even slightly higher protein partly due to the increased satiety.

It is important to note though that when you are in a calorie deficit, it may be beneficial to increase protein intake beyond what you may eat when maintaining.

This increase in protein may not only help with muscle retention, but lead to faster weight loss!

A higher protein ratio will also force you to dial in the overall quality of your food in many cases.

And if you're familiar with bodybuilding calculations...

A standard bodybuilding recommendation is to get about 1 gram per pound of bodyweight, which is usually about 40% of your total calories.

Studies of high protein diets have even looked at diets where protein is 4.4 grams per kg of bodyweight or about 2 grams per pound of bodyweight and have shown no negative health effects and also no fat gain when eating in a calorie surplus!

The exact amount of protein you decide to include may be based on your goals, workouts and even your age with a higher protein ratio especially benefiting you if you are looking to really get that six pack!

As you begin to plan to eat according to your goals, I'll provide some ranges you can work in based on the results you want to achieve and even the LENGTH of time you'll be sticking with a ratio.

Because when we are driving to kickstart weight loss results versus maintaining our current weight, the amount we need of each macro may change!

But Isn't A High Protein Diet Dangerous?

When making any dietary changes, you always want to consult a doctor if you have specific health issues or illnesses. Because then, yes, a variety of diets may be detrimental.

But unless you have a specific health concern?

High protein diets are not only safe, but they may actually be the key to improving your health!

The conditions people fear a high protein diet may put them at risk for are:
-Osteoporosis
-Cardiovascular disease
-Kidney damage

But these fears are unfounded for healthy individuals.

While you may want to watch your protein intake if you have kidney disease or kidney stones already, in healthy individuals, studies have shown no increased risk of kidney damage with an extremely high protein intake.

Now what about your bone health? Can high protein leach minerals from your bones and cause osteoporosis as was once believed?

NOPE!

Bones are made up of protein yet for awhile the "myth" existed that a high protein diet was bad for your bones.

But the exact opposite is actually true.

High protein diets can help improve bone density and prevent osteoporosis. The amino acids in protein are used to build bone and because protein increases muscles mass, there is also an increase in bone strength!

Studies have even started looking at whether or not we need to INCREASE our protein recommendations further for older adults to help prevent an increased occurrence of fractures.

And what about cardiovascular disease? Is protein bad for your cholesterol and heart health?

No! Actually it may improve indicators of cardiometabolic health, including lowering blood pressure and IMPROVING blood cholesterol.

But the QUALITY of your protein sources matters!

Consuming crap or junk food isn't ideal for your health no matter what macro it's made up of.

So if you want to keep your heart healthy, consume healthy and whole, natural sources of protein. Eat more seafood. Choose naturally raised animal protein sources. Even get extra amino acids from plant sources.

Consume QUALITY protein and you'll help keep your body healthy!

And finally…what about kidney damage?

If you have kidney issues or a history of kidney stones, you NEED to consult your doctor before making any dietary changes, especially increasing protein.

And because low protein diets have been recommended in the past to people with kidney disease, the myth grew that high protein diets were bad for the kidneys.

But it's like telling someone with no injuries not to run just because you shouldn't run with a broken leg.

While running on a broken leg may cause overload and further injury, running is in no way bad for the overall health of an individual.

And while high protein diets do cause your kidneys to work more, it's the same thing as running causing your legs to work more than when you walk. It's not harmful unless you already have that broken leg!

Studies have even looked at diets with extremely high protein intakes and shown no negative effects on healthy kidneys even when these diets have been done for extended periods of time.

It is recommended though that you increase your water intake to avoid dehydration when increasing your protein intake.

The Complete Health Benefits Of Protein - Let's Also Talk About MICROnutrients

Most often high protein diets are talked about for weight loss or even gaining muscle.

But they have health benefits as well!

As I've mentioned, a diet higher in protein can help us increase our bone density, recover from injury and stay active and mobile as we get older.

Protein not only makes up all of our tissues, which is why it is important for our bone and muscle health, but it also helps carry the oxygen that reddens our blood, combines with sterols to form hormones and is needed for the transport of fat and cholesterol throughout our bodies.

This means that getting more protein can help improve brain functioning, quality of sleep AND lower blood pressure!

Newer studies are being done on the impact higher protein intakes have on our cognitive functioning as we get older. There seems to be promise that a higher protein diet may have benefit in helping prevent Alzheimer's disease.

But it isn't just protein in general that is good for our health.

Often when we dial in the ratios of our macronutrients, we also benefit by getting more of the MICROnutrients we need.

When we think micronutrients we often think about eating more fruits and veggies. But protein sources are jammed pack with essential micronutrients that often go unrecognized.

There are different types of each vitamin that need to be consumed from different sources, which is why VARIETY IS KEY in our diets.

And while we don't often think of protein as something we "need" for our health outside of the amino acids as building blocks, it can be an important source of many vitamins and minerals that aren't available in the same form elsewhere!

Some important vitamins and minerals we get from protein sources are:

-Vitamin A can be found in eggs, liver and fish
-Vitamin B12 can be found in fish, meat and eggs
-Iodine can be found in fish
-Iron can be found in red meat, poultry and fish
-Zinc can be found in liver, eggs and seafood
-Vitamin D3 can be found in fatty fish and egg yolks.
-Vitamin D3, or cholecalciferol, is found in animals and is much more potent than ergocalciferol (or vitamin D2 found in plants). (By "potent," I mean it increases blood levels of vitamin D more efficiently.)

There are also ANTIOXIDANTS such as carnosine in meat and fish.

Carnosine is important for muscle function and high levels in muscle tissue have been linked to reduced muscle fatigue and improved performance.

Docosahexaenoic acid (DHA), also found mainly in fatty fish and fish oil, is an essential omega-3 fatty acid and essential to normal brain development and functioning.

The point is...there are tons of different HEALTH benefits found in these protein sources.

Even minerals we think we NEED from fruits and veggies can be found as well in animal protein.

For instance...POTASSIUM!

A boneless pork loin chop, for instance, has about 770 milligrams, which is 16% of your daily intake.

And chicken not only has potassium, but also magnesium and calcium.

Plus, we have to note that different TYPES of each vitamin, take for instance vitamin K, need to be gotten from different sources.

Vitamin K1 may be gotten from plant AND animal sources while vitamin K2 comes from animal sources. While we can make K2 from K1, it isn't fully enough.

The point of this isn't to convince you to eat meat, but to show you that VARIETY CAN BE KEY!

And that by focusing on increasing the protein in your diet, you can also get many of the micronutrients you need!

The point is that we often ONLY consider fruits and vegetables and not all of the whole, natural foods out there and their health benefits.

And that's why we need all sorts of whole, natural foods, and a wide variety, to really meet our needs.

But What If I Don't Eat Meat?

While animal protein does contain a variety of vitamins and minerals we need, that doesn't mean you have to consume animal sources to get enough protein.

I know that when we think of protein, we think of meat.
But you can get protein from plant sources if you don't choose to consume animal products!

It is key though that we understand the difference between "complete" amino acid chains and "incomplete" amino acid chains.

While you don't need to eat meat to get enough protein, you do want to understand that you may need to COMBINE amino acid sources from different vegetables, grains, legumes, seeds, beans and nuts to create a full amino acid chain.

There are about 13 nonessential and 9 essential amino acids. These essential amino acids are what affect whether or not a protein is considered complete.

A complete protein has all 9 essential amino acids in sufficient quantities to help us meet our body's needs.

And, yes, animal proteins are complete proteins. Meat, fish and eggs are all complete protein sources.

So is dairy, and not only milk and yogurt, but also the derivatives often made into protein powders aka WHEY.

There are also NON-animal sources of complete proteins including:

-Quinoa
-Buckwheat
-Soy (tofu and tempeh)

Chia seeds and hemp seeds are ALMOST complete proteins as well but are too low in lysine to fully qualify.

Incomplete proteins, on the other hand, don't necessarily have all 9 essential amino acids or don't have enough of them to meet our body's needs so we need to supplement them with other proteins.

This doesn't mean these protein sources are in any way bad or "worse" just that we need to combine foods to meet our needs.

These combinations of amino acid sources are called complementary proteins and include combinations such as:

31

-Rice and beans
-Spinach and almonds (say in a salad)
-Chickpeas and whole-grains (say hummus and pitas)
-Whole-grains and peanuts (say peanut butter on whole grain bread)
-Legumes and grains (combined in say soups or stews)
-Spirulina with grains or nuts

The combination of these foods together provides us with sufficient quantities of all 9 essential amino acids. But while they need to be combined, they don't need to be eaten right together, but just eaten throughout the day's meals.

And of course, there are protein supplements you can include from whey and casein (if you aren't Vegan) to rice and pea and even egg white (again if you aren't Vegan).

Collagen is also another option to increase your protein intake although it does come from animal sources. If you are a pescatarian, this can be a great option as they do have ones from fish.

If you do choose to use a protein supplement, combining even pea and rice protein TOGETHER can create a killer source of protein too!

As long as you get adequate amounts of amino acids to support proper body functioning, all sources of protein can and should be included.

The more variety you can include in your diet, the better.

Even if you are a meat eater, including more vegetables, or plant-based sources of protein, can be key to improving your health AND making your diet more enjoyable!

Just be conscious, if you don't eat meat, that you are getting all 9 essential amino acids in high enough quantities!

Let's Talk About Carbs:

Carb-phobia is real.

And all too often carbs are demonized when they don't need to be, especially when it comes to weight loss.

Because cutting carbs...well it leads to pretty instant "results" on the scale.

It's what I call "fake weight loss" because you haven't actually lost any fat, yet the scale number will go down pretty quickly.

So if this weight loss isn't "real," what are we losing instantly with a low carb diet?

When you change to a low carb diet, two things happen:

You deplete your glycogen stores, which results in weight loss.

You lose water weight.

And neither one of these things is necessarily bad, BUT they are why the scale can fluctuate so much and you may find the second you "cheat," or have a higher carb meal, all of the weight comes right back.

Because for every gram of glycogen your body stores (which glycogen storage isn't necessarily a bad thing!), comes with it about 3-4 grams of water.

Basically you can go on a low carb diet and deplete your glycogen stores to lose 6.6lbs or about 3kg pretty freaking instantly.

So going lower carb can be a way to see very fast, albeit not necessarily "true," results.

But exactly how many carbs you need to consume will be impacted by any health issues you may have, your goals and even your training and overall activity level.

Carbs are NOT evil though and actually eating too few, while it may have initially helped, may be hindering you from making further progress.

So What Are Carbs?

Carbs are organic molecules that, based on their structure, can be broken down into two different types - simple and complex.

Simple carbs have one or two sugar molecules linked together and are smaller and more easily processed by the body. They are known as monosaccharides or disaccharides.

Complex carbs all have more than two sugar molecules linked together and are called polysaccharides. If they have 3-10 units of sugar linked, they can be called oligosaccharides.

Oligosaccharides are short chains of monosaccharide units while polysaccharides are long chains of monosaccharide units put together.

Simple and complex carbs BOTH have their place and use, but often you'll hear that simple carbs are bad for you and complex carbs are good - that's if we're eating carbs at all.

And it's important to understand that ALL carbs are broken down in our bodies into monosaccharides, or simple sugars, before being used.

The difference really is how quickly these carbs are digested and absorbed with complex carbs being absorbed more slowly. However, the other foods we consume with carbs can change the rate of digestion and absorption.

But regardless of the type, carbs, simple and complex, are an immediate source of energy for all of the body's cells.

Why Are Carbs Important?

For some people, lower carb simply WILL be better.

If you are very sedentary and/or just starting to lose weight, you may find lower carb works well for you, especially at the start of your journey.

And there are some people that are metabolically adapted to handle fat better than they do carbs.

Even certain diseases and illnesses mean going lower carb to alleviate symptoms.

But it is key you don't just instantly demonize a macro because that fear of carbs may be holding you back, ESPECIALLY if you train intensely!

It is important that you understand the role carbs plays in your body so you can see how they can help, or hurt, you.

So what functions do carbs contribute to in our bodies?

Carbs play an integral role in keeping our hormones at optimal levels - specifically T3, cortisol and testosterone levels.

T3 is a thyroid hormone that helps us maintain proper metabolic function and is important for blood glucose management.

When our carb intake drops, our levels of T3 decrease and our levels of Reverse T3, which further inhibits T3 from working, increase.

This can not only hinder our weight loss results, but can also negatively impact our energy levels and, therefore, the results we get from our workouts.

Thyroid hormone problems can also lead to anxiety issues and contribute to menstrual irregularities (aka missed periods!).

These issues can be compounded by a calorie deficit while training hard on lower carb.

If you're working out or more active, and especially if you're working out more intensely, carbs are even more important than you may realize.

While we often think about the important role that protein plays in muscle retention and building lean muscle, carbs also play an important role in this process! They can help us avoid muscle catabolism and even assist in creating an anabolic environment, which is essential to promoting muscle growth!

If our carb intake drops too low for our needs, we may even fight against our gains no matter how much protein we consume.

How do carbs help us retain and build lean muscle?

When we consume enough carbs, especially if we are exercising regularly, we can keep our testosterone, and other anabolic hormone levels higher and our cortisol levels lower. Basically we create hormone levels that PROMOTE muscle growth.

While if we cut carbs too low, our testosterone will drop and our cortisol levels will rise. This can lead to not only muscle loss, but us gaining fat.

Consuming a very low carb diet may also lead to muscle loss due to a drop in insulin levels.

While many of us have heard that higher insulin levels are bad, insulin is not this horrible thing we need to fear and actually plays a crucial role in building muscle. Again, too often we completely demonize things that have a role to play in our body (even cortisol isn't something to be completely feared).

Especially when you're training hard, you need to replenish your muscle glycogen to create an anabolic hormonal environment and grow that muscle!

If you don't consume enough carbs, you're going to actually create an environment that not only leads to less protein synthesis (so less muscle growth no matter how much protein you consume), but also muscle catabolism.

So if you're working hard to build muscle in the gym, you need to consume enough carbs to see results.

Consuming too few carbs can also negatively impact our performance.

And let's face it, if you aren't progressing in your training, you're probably going to be getting lackluster results even though you feel like you're working hard and pushing yourself in the gym!

Carbs also play an important role in proper cognitive functioning, mood regulation and a healthy immune system!

And ladies? We can be more sensitive to changes in our carb intake.

While organs, like our thyroid, make hormones, our hormone production system is controlled by our central nervous system and our BRAIN.

Our hypothalamus and pituitary glands sit in our brain and are sensitive to changes in energy availability and our stress level. (While it's a good stressor, exercise can impact our stress levels!)

Both the hypothalamus and pituitary glands work together with our adrenal glands in a partnership known as the hypothalamic-pituitary-adrenal, or HPA, axis.

The HPA axis regulates functions including our:

-Stress response
-Mood
-Digestion
-Immune system
-Libido
-Metabolism
-And even our energy levels

Because this system is so sensitive to stress and energy availability, going low carb may have a negative impact and even more of one on women who may be more sensitive to changes in their carb intake while working out intensely.

The result of going low carb and disrupting proper functioning of our HPA axis may be hypothalamic amenorrhea - irregular or stopped periods due to a disruption in hormone levels.

And while not eating enough calories can also be a cause, you can still suffer from a disruption in your hormone balance simply by not eating enough carbs even if you're technically consuming enough calories!

Because a low carb intake can also cause an increase in cortisol levels, this can also signal the HPA axis to further decrease pituitary activity. And the pituitary gland, in particular, is responsible for synthesizing and secreting growth hormone, a thyroid stimulating hormone and other incredibly important hormones.

So making sure to get enough carbs is ESSENTIAL to maintaining optimal hormone levels, especially for women who train hard!

But how much is "enough" and what really constitutes low carb?

What Really Constitutes Low Carb?

Low carb can mean a variety of different things to different people.

And our personal needs will differ affecting what is specifically "too low" for us.

Not only are some of us more carb or fat adapted, meaning our metabolism naturally responds better to carbs or fat as fuel, but we have different goals, activity levels and even health issues that may affect our needs.

This is why it can be helpful to start by alternating ratios every few weeks, but specifically alternating ratios of higher or lower carb to see which seems to fit best. This can help you determine what is too high or too low for you.

But to give a range, for the healthy moderately active individual, under 100 grams of carbs, about 10-15% of your calories coming from carbs, is considered "low carb" while under 50 grams, or 10% or less, is considered necessary for some with specific health issues or to enter ketosis.

Under 50 grams of carbs is really only recommended for those with metabolic syndrome or even for those with neurological issues or severe blood sugar problems. Please make sure to consult your doctor if you do have an issue you feel may be helped by a lower carb diet before making any dramatic dietary changes.

While a low carb intake of 10% or less has become more popular recently for weight loss due to the rise of Keto, it is key we recognize this is an aggressive and short-term strategy for most people. And it is probably best suited to those who are inactive and almost completely sedentary with 100lbs or more to lose.

But for most of the population, under 50 grams of carbs is NOT sustainable nor necessary to achieve results. It almost makes getting lasting results more difficult.

Even bumping your carb intake to just between 10-15% of your calories will still be on the aggressive side, leading to the fast weight loss people often seek from a low carb diet with less risk of throwing your hormones out of balance. We also have to remember that the quick drop in weight we often see from going low carb isn't true fat loss, but instead our glycogen stores being depleted and water weight being lost.

And this range can also be good for anyone with blood sugar regulation issues or digestion issues due to certain types of carbs.

If you are a generally healthy and active individual, a carb intake between 15-30% will most likely be right for you. This range will still allow you to lose weight but can also be a range you stay in to maintain your weight after your goal is achieved.

Cutting our carbs super low often backfires, leading to us regaining the weight because we can't maintain that low intake forever. If instead we create a diet with a carb intake we can stick to, we'll set ourselves up for long-term success!

Also, if you do have hypothyroidism, or an underactive thyroid, a carb intake of between 15-30% of your daily calorie needs is generally low enough to help you lose weight while still staying fueled!

And if you are a super active person with a fast metabolism, an endurance athlete, breastfeeding or trying to gain muscle, you may find you actually increase your carb intake to between 30-50% of your daily caloric intake.

Remember, carbs play a key role in keeping us energized while helping us to maintain optimal hormone levels and prevent muscle catabolism.

"Good" Vs. "Bad" Carbs

As you figure out how many carbs you need based on your needs and goals, you also need to consider the TYPE of carbs you consume.

While processed food is never ideal, we don't want to label foods as "good" or "bad" because this can lead to guilt when we consume foods on that "bad" list.

And even what foods may be "good" or "bad" for you may be based on your goals, health issues or dietary preference.

Let's take for example GLUTEN.

If you have a gluten intolerance, if you have Celiac disease, you're going to need to avoid gluten. Plain and simple.

But if you don't have an intolerance to it, you don't have to demonize it and cut it out.

Even digestion issues or other food sensitivities may require you to cut out specific foods. But this doesn't mean foods are evil. It just means they aren't right for YOU.

Some of these sensitivities may even require you to cut out so called "healthy" carb sources.

For instance, if you have IBS and start eliminating foods high in FODMAPs, you may end up finding you are sensitive to asparagus, brussel sprouts or even BROCCOLI! And these vegetables are nutrient-dense and often

37

touted as healthy!

So it is key we not only look for nutrient-dense carbs, but also focus on finding sources that make us feel good!

Now what about glycemic index...Aren't higher glycemic index foods bad?

Yes and no.

Sure processed cereals, corn syrup and other processed and refined grains aren't ideal. They are devoid of many essential nutrients we need.

And specific health issues such as diabetes may mean paying attention to the glycemic index of the foods you eat.

But just because something is fairly high on the glycemic index doesn't mean it's bad!

There are some amazing fruits and even starchy vegetables higher on the glycemic index that are nutrient dense, such as the sweet potato!

These high glycemic index foods may even have their place in your diet if you're training hard and trying to maximize muscle hypertrophy while staying lean.

Especially when striving for specific performance or aesthetic goals, timing some simple carbs post workout may BENEFIT you!

The key thing to remember is you want to include as many NUTRIENT-DENSE carbs as possible.

Focus your diet on fruits and vegetables while including a range of other carbs based on your training goals and health needs.

But don't feel like you can't also indulge in some of those less nutritionally dense carbs you love too. Just focus on 80% of your foods coming from whole, natural sources!

Consuming a variety of different carb sources allows us to get the vitamins and minerals we need while keeping our meals enjoyable!

Who Does Lower Carb Work Better For?

Adjusting your carb intake can help you work toward different goals based on your specific needs and activity level.

If you are super sedentary and not working out, a lower carb intake may be ideal. You simply don't need the instant fuel that carbs provide.

A lower carb intake may also be more beneficial for someone with 70 or more pounds to lose who is just starting their weight loss journey. When we dramatically cut back on carbs that restriction of a macro can help create a calorie deficit to provide faster results and added motivation.

A lower carb macro breakdown, may be used strategically as a kickstart to help you get the ball rolling and see progress in the right direction.

It may also be used toward the end of a cut if you are striving for specific physique goals and need a little kickstart but don't want to drop your calories any lower.

Especially if you are looking to make a dietary change for health reasons, you may determine that a lower carb macro ratio is the way to go for you. It is key you discuss these changes with your doctor, but it is good to learn when adjusting your diet could help so you can start a discussion!

For instance, low carb diets, specifically Keto, have shown promise when it comes to helping alleviate the symptoms of certain health issues. A dietary change to a lower carb intake may help with treatment of specific symptoms.

While Keto has risen in popularity as a diet for weight loss, it was actually originally tested and created to help people with epilepsy and seizures.

While it may not PREVENT these issues from occurring in the first place, it has been shown to help with "treatment" or management of them.

I think it is key here to also note that Keto and low carb are not necessarily one in the same.

While Keto or the Ketogenic Diet is a low carb diet, not all low carb diets are Keto.

The extremely low carb ratios of Keto have also been shown to decrease inflammation and help with Alzheimer's, metabolic syndrome and potentially even help patients with cancer.

So for people with these health issues, trying a Keto, or extremely low carb, diet may be beneficial BUT studies haven't proven it will PREVENT these health conditions.

If you DON'T have a health issue, these extremely low carb intakes may lead to initial weight loss results, and even make you feel better initial, but could end up being detrimental long term.

Especially if you are more active, carbs are ESSENTIAL to getting results and important for maintaining hormonal balance.

Cutting your carbs too low, while it may initially seem like it's providing you with fast results, will end up holding you back the more active you are. Especially if you're female.

Not only can it cause hormonal imbalances, but your performance will suffer AND you may end up actually GAINING belly fat!

Yup! Cutting your carbs too low may end up hindering your fat loss progress.

If you are more active, you may want to stick with a carb intake between 15-30% of your calories. This is still "lower carb," and can even work well for those more metabolically fat adapted (aka you run "better" off of fat) while still fueling your activity!

Just remember, carbs are NOT evil. While people fear consuming carbs may make them gain belly fat, that simply isn't the case (and again, under consuming carbs may actually have that exact effect you're trying to avoid).

Carbs are key to help our body function properly.

Just remember that if you regularly exercise intensely, and cut your carbs too low, you can end up causing the following issues to occur:

-A suppressed immune system
-Muscle loss
-Irregular or stopped periods
-Mood swings (and oddly enough blood sugar swings)
-Bone density loss
-Increased feelings of anxiety and depression
-Increased inflammation
-Disrupted sleep
-Brain fog

Remember, our carb intake should be based on our needs and our activity level!

Let's Talk About Fat:

Let's get one thing straight right now...Eating fat does NOT make you fat.

A product that says "Low-Fat" isn't automatically healthy...and may actually even be worse than the full fat alternative.

While fat is our primary form of energy storage, eating fat does not automatically make us store fat.

We store fat because we overeat and eat a diet that isn't balanced.

We can also store fat because our body is in a bit of a "crisis" from under eating or from stress (not only daily stress from work and family life but even over exercising).

Not getting enough healthy fats in our diet can contribute to, and perpetuate, that "crisis" and end up leading to a whole host of health problems.

While fats can be a source of fuel for our body, they are also crucial to our health and a diet rich in healthy fats helps our body function optimally.

However, your overall fat intake will vary based on how fat adapted you are and even your goals.

Especially for more aesthetic based goals, like getting a six pack, lower fat intakes may be key.

Because it can be detrimental to drop your fat intake too low for too long, it can be important to cycle in some higher fat ratios.

We need to stop just demonizing a macro because not only does each macro play a role in helping our body function properly, BUT there are healthier, and less healthy, sources of each macronutrient that do impact the benefits we reap from them!

By dialing in our macros we can even improve our training to speed up our results while optimizing our recovery!

YUP! A macro ratio that helps you stay fueled and promotes optimal body functioning will help you sleep better and recover faster!

So What Are Fats?

Fats, also called lipids, are organic molecules that consist mainly of carbon and hydrogen elements. They are joined together into long chains called hydrocarbons and may, or may not, be joined together by a double bond.

The configuration of these molecules creates different types of fats and gives them their unique properties.

Basically, the way the molecules are constructed will determine the type of fat they are - saturated, monounsaturated or polyunsaturated fat.

There is also trans fat, which can be artificially made. And artificial trans fat has been shown to increase the risk of heart disease, cancer, obesity and overall inflammation that can lead to disease.

Each of these types of fat play a different role in our body.

And while monounsaturated fat is the only truly "agreed upon" healthy fat across a variety of dietary preferences (with omega-3s, a type of polyunsaturated fat, gaining in popularity), saturated, polyunsaturated and even natural trans fats all play an important role in keeping us healthy and helping us achieve our dietary goals!

Why Are Fats Important?

While you have those people that believe consuming carbs will make them gain belly fat, you also have those people that believe fat will make them fat.

When, in fact, consuming enough healthy fat may actually aid your weight loss efforts!

From keeping our hormone levels in balance to simply keeping us feeling fuller and more satisfied between meals, consuming enough fat in our diet is key if we want to lose weight.

Getting enough fat can also keep our joints healthy, which can help us get more out of our workouts.

And in terms of health benefits, healthy fats are essential because they:

-Support a healthy metabolism
-Promote proper absorption of vitamins A, D, E and K
-Preserve your eye health
-Promote hormone production
-Support a healthy immune system

-Maintain healthy brain functioning
-Promote optimal cell signaling
-Keep tissues such as your skin and hair healthy

We need to especially focus on getting more omega-3s in our diet as improving our ratio of omega-3s to omega-6s may be the key to reducing inflammation in our bodies. Inflammation not only fights against our weight loss and fat loss efforts but can be a leading cause of disease!

So the types of fats you consume can really make a difference!

What Really Is A "Healthy" Fat?

If you want the best results possible, you want to focus on consuming as many whole, natural, nutrient-dense foods as you can.

And while I firmly believe we need to end this "clean eating" obsession, because it only leads to guilt when we indulge, let's face it…

Processed foods are not good for us.

So logically it does make sense that processed fats wouldn't be good for us either.

For instance, while natural trans fats may have some health benefits, we want to avoid its artificial counterpart at all costs.

What foods contain this processed trans fat?

Vegetable oils (canola, soybean and corn oil), margarines, vegetable shortening…even some non-dairy creamers have trans fat when they say they don't.

Even most fried and processed foods, including many of the baked goods we consume (especially those with basically no expiration date), contain trans fat.

Artificial trans fat not only doesn't provide us with any benefits, but it has actually been shown to be detrimental to our health.

Even with relatively small doses, artificial trans fats have been shown to increase our risk of cancer, heart disease and obesity. They may also increase inflammation in our body, leading to other inflammatory conditions such as metabolic syndrome or even arthritis.

Now…what about naturally occurring fats?

Aren't some of those bad as well?

This is where discussions can get heated because the only really agreed upon "healthy" fats are monounsaturated fats. However, omega-3s are also extremely important and are rising in "popularity" as a healthy fat.

Monounsaturated fats are found in foods like olives, nuts, seeds and avocados.

They've been shown to be beneficial for heart health and may reduce the risk for heart disease, lowering LDL and triglycerides while potentially increasing HDL. They've also been shown to help decrease oxidized LDL, reduce inflammation and lower blood pressure.

Omega-3s, which are a type of polyunsaturated fat, have also been shown to have great health benefits.

There are 6 types of omega-3s, but 3 we often focus on as the most important.

One omega-3, ALA or Alpha-linoleic acid, can be found in plant foods such as walnuts and flax seeds.

While the other two, EPA, or Eicosapentaenoic acid, and DHA, or Docosahexaenoic acid, can be found in fatty cold-water fish, such as salmon, sardines, mackerel and bass as well shellfish, like oysters and mussels.

Omega-3s have been shown to reduce our risk of several chronic inflammatory diseases, including coronary heart disease.

DHA is also essential for proper brain development and getting enough DHA may help us maintain healthy brain functioning even as we get older!

But it isn't just about getting more omega-3s in our diet.

It is also about paying attention to our intake of omega-6s.

But the answer isn't as simple as don't eat omega-6s because these not only naturally occur in some of the "healthy" foods we eat, but are also necessary for our body to function properly.

We will find forms of omega-6s in some of the fruits, vegetables, meats and even nuts and seeds we eat.

Our body does need these omega-6s from whole, natural sources to function properly.

Omega-6s can help maintain proper cellular signaling and even help maintain healthy blood pressure. They can also assist in proper muscle growth and repair.

What we DO need to pay attention to is the ratio of omega-3s to omega-6s.

While ideally we want to shoot for a 1:1 ratio of omega-6s to omega-3s, often now the ratio we see in people's diets is 10:1 to 20:1.

And this ratio, and the excess omega-6s, is what can lead to inflammation as well as weight gain, liver disease, cancer, autoimmune diseases and even premature aging.

We see this imbalanced ratio occurring, not because of the whole natural sources we are consuming (although grass-fed and naturally raised animals will give you a far better ratio of omega-3s to omega-6s) but because we are consuming far too many omega-6s from processed foods.

Industrially processed and refined seed oils such as soybean, cottonseed, corn, safflower and sunflower oils all contribute to our excess omega-6 intake. So do many of the cereals we consume.

Again, whole, natural foods are key!

The one NATURALLY occurring fat source that is often demonized though is saturated fat because studies have linked it to an increased risk of heart disease.

Saturated fat is found in basically all animal products, from meat to eggs and dairy.

Recent studies have called into question these findings showing that lower carb diets higher in saturated fat may actually have a beneficial impact on several markers of cardiovascular disease including triglyceride levels, fasting glucose, blood pressure, HDL cholesterol, c-reactive protein and more.

So if you follow a lower carb diet ratio, or even a Paleo dietary preference, you may find you do consume more saturated fat without any negative impact to your health.

The key is also realizing you don't necessarily need to fear saturated fat as long as you consume a diet rich in monounsaturated fats and omega-3s!

How Much Fat Do You Really Need?

Some extremely low fat diets put fat intake at about 10% of your daily calorie intake.
This low fat intake is not a sustainable, long-term solution.

Dropping your fat intake this low for extended periods of time may lead to hormonal imbalances and nutrient deficiencies.

While a macro breakdown with only 10% of your calories coming from fat may be used as a kickstart or a final cut for someone in a physique competition, it is key to note this is a more extreme ratio and meant for a short-term fix or purpose.

However, if you are more carb-adapted and want to lose weight and fat, you can still follow a lower fat ratio while maintaining healthy bodily functioning with between 15-20% of your calories coming from fat.

Studies have shown this intake to be sufficient even if weight loss is your goal and you are in a calorie deficit.

If you are female and looking to go lower fat, not dropping below 15% will help you maintain proper reproductive functioning.

Endurance athletes may also use lower fat ratios, keeping their fat intake between 15-20%. This can help as they increase carbs to fuel their training while keeping protein as high as possible to prevent muscle catabolism.

For many of us though, staying between 20-35% of our calories coming from fat can lead to great aesthetic results, including fat loss, while promoting optimal health and energy levels.

Around 30% fat is often where we settle to maintain our results and build a lifestyle.

However, if you choose to do a lower carb ratio, your fat intake will go above 35%. This is where you start to

44

creep into higher fat ratios. And that is not a bad thing. You'll just want to have the extra grams of fat come from your carb intake over your protein intake.

Usually with lower carb ratios, fat intakes will be between 40-60% of your daily intake. Some more extreme low carb diets will even bump fat toward 70%.

Just remember when we go to either extreme, either really slashing carbs or fat, it may be a short-term solution but we have to be conscious of the potential effects to our health!

Who Does A Low Fat Diet Work Best For?

Fat will NOT make you fat. And a higher fat macronutrient breakdown can help you lose weight, especially if you are less active or metabolically more fat-adapted (aka you naturally run better off of fat).

But if you're more active and looking to reach lower levels of leanness, maybe even achieving a six pack for the first time, lower fat ratios may be ideal.

Lower fat ratios can also be key when trying to gain muscle. Carbs help us gain muscle by promoting an anabolic environment in our body and by helping create an environment more conducive to recovery.

When you restrict carbs, your muscle glycogen levels drop and low glycogen stores can inhibit signaling related to post-workout muscle repair and growth.

Also, since you will be training hard, restricting your carbs can raise cortisol levels and lower testosterone levels which will also affect recovery.

Low carb diets can also decrease strength and muscular endurance, making it harder to create progressive overload in your workouts, which will hinder maximal muscle growth.

For this reason, going lower fat so you can focus on carbs is key!

Now for weight loss, both low fat and low carb can honestly work. What it comes down to is your activity level, what you tend to crave the most and also how fat or carb adapted you are.

Even the mental satisfaction you get from eating certain foods and portions can play a role!

It's important to note that while fat can make you feel fuller for longer between meals, which can be helpful for weight loss, its caloric density can also backfire.

Fat has 9 calories per gram compared to the 4 calories per gram in both protein and carbs.

With over double the calories per gram, fat calories can add up quickly.

When we are in a calorie deficit especially, there is a certain satisfaction to eating a greater quantity of food.

It's why eating more vegetables can be key! They are nutritionally dense and less calorically dense so you get to eat a larger quantity, which can also make you feel full and satisfied.

Whereas if you were to eat nuts, a high fat food, as a snack, you only get to eat a very small serving and a few bites.

It is often easier to overeat fats, which can not only throw off your macro ratio, but kick you out of the calorie deficit you need to be in to lose weight.

So going lower fat may work best for you just because you can eat a larger quantity of food!

You may also want to vary your fat intake based on where you are in your weight loss journey.

While protein's thermic effect is much more constant regardless of your current body composition, studies have shown that fat's thermic effect may actually be LOWER in obese individuals.

This means you're not going to get any extra calorie burn from consuming more fat if you're obese, which alone isn't a reason to go low fat.

But if you are starting a workout routine as you begin your weight loss journey, meaning you'll no longer be as sedentary, you may want to consider cycling in a lower fat ratio every few weeks to get the added benefit of the higher thermic effect of protein and carbs.

If you are leaner, and even looking to maintain your leanness, you may be able to go slightly higher in fat as you'll then get the small thermic effect that fat offers.

If You Can Only Focus On One Macro….

The best diet is the one you can stick to.

And you may find you cycle between higher fat and higher carb ratios, especially as your lifestyle or workouts change.

The one constant there needs to be is a focus on protein.

There are studies proving that both high fat and high carb diets can work for weight loss.

The one flaw with most of these studies is that protein is never held constant.

The diet that always comes out on top in the study being performed is also always the diet that is higher in protein.

So if you are just starting out, and not sure if higher carb or higher fat will work best, focus first on protein.

Studies have even shown that higher protein diets give you more "wiggle room," aka you can technically be in a caloric surplus, without gaining body fat.

Now this isn't an excuse to overeat just because you're eating more protein, but it does show you that by dialing in your macros correctly, and focusing on them first, you can get great results without having to worry about strictly eating a very specific calorie intake.

By focusing on protein first, we can then adjust our carb and fat intake off of what we find we enjoy more, how our energy levels feel, our workouts as they change over time and even what we personally respond best to!

Food Quality: Why It Does…And Doesn't…Matter

Food quality matters not only for your health, but also for achieving your aesthetic and performance goals faster and more efficiently.

Let's face it…processed food isn't good for you and whole, natural foods fuel you better.

However, all too often we start eating "healthy foods" yet don't see the long-term weight loss, or fat loss, results we want.

We may initially see results from eliminating foods, or even whole food groups, because that automatically often cuts our calories, but generally those results slow or completely stall before we've reached our ultimate goal.

And this is because, while quality matters, it also doesn't matter.

We can still overeat even eating whole natural foods. (Especially often those fatty snacks we turn to like nuts.)

We can still eat a macro breakdown that isn't focused on our goals and doesn't match our energy demands.

It's why if you have a specific performance or aesthetic goal, you need to focus on hitting those macro ratios and calories FIRST as you adjust your food choices to match.

Because by focusing on hitting your macro ratios, you WILL also dial in the overall quality of your food without feeling like anything necessarily has to be off limits.

You can still indulge in those foods you love.

And, over time, as you adjust to the changes, it can be easier and easier to adjust your food quality, focusing more and more on whole, natural foods that will give you the micronutrients you also need.

Even if the sole focus of our diet is improving our health, we need to stop demonizing foods and labeling them as "good" and "bad."

We need to stop this pressure to "eat clean." We need to stop making foods "off limits."

We need to avoid these strict elimination diets that make us feel bad for eating even specific vegetables and fruits!

Because achieving results isn't about perfection, it's about consistency.

And what helps us be the most consistent is a balance of doing what we know we should to achieve results with enjoying and indulging and relaxing at times too.

Too often a restrictive attitude holds us back. And guilt is what derails us.

Plus, improving your health means REDUCING the negative stressors on your body, not adding to them!

Eating according to your goals shouldn't make you feel more stressed out. It should enhance your life.

While yes, initially changes can be stressful and even feel overwhelming, your diet shouldn't make you more obsessed about food because you're trying so hard to avoid certain things.

Because when you devote your whole life to completely avoiding something, that thing will still end up controlling your life!

Food is fuel. BUT food can also be social and fun and we shouldn't have to give that up.

It is about finding a balance.

This means recognizing that while we do want to focus our diet on quality fuel, we should not be obsessing over eating "clean."

It also means realizing that what is considered a "clean" food is not universally agreed upon across a variety of dietary preferences. If you choose to go Paleo vs. Vegetarian vs. Traditional, "clean" means so many different things.

So focusing your diet about 80% of the time on whole, natural foods, that are grown with the best farming practices possible, is key.

And then 20% of the time, indulge in the not so healthy treats you also enjoy so you can find a balance!

The Benefit Of Whole, Natural Foods

If you dial in your macros and maintain a calorie deficit, you will lose weight. EVEN if you're eating a diet full of processed foods.

Is this necessarily a good thing?

No.

BUT it's still us making a positive change - it's still a step in the right direction.

And for some, it may be where we need to start to get the ball rolling.

However, ideally, yes, we want to try to follow the 80/20 rule, consuming 80% of our calories from whole, natural food sources.

Because whole, natural foods DO actually help us get better aesthetic and performance results, whether we want to lose weight, gain muscle, achieve that six pack or even fuel our sport.

I know we often focus on "quality" for our health, but there are a few different ways that healthy foods benefit us when working toward these other goals!

And one of those benefits we can get from whole, natural foods is a higher thermic effect!

Whole, natural foods require you to burn more calories to digest them than processed foods, which will help you get better results faster, especially if weight loss is your goal or if you want to stay leaner as you gain muscle.

Something even as simple as switching your sandwich from processed white bread and fake cheese to whole grain bread and natural cheese can make a difference!

And that isn't even really making that dramatic a quality change!

Not only do whole, natural foods have a higher thermic effect, but they also help us feel fuller for longer even when in a deficit.

Whole, natural foods allow us to consume a larger volume of food, while consuming far fewer calories, than most of the processed foods we often reach for.

This alone can make whole, natural foods more satisfying even when we consume far fewer calories. There is something about simply the VOLUME of food you get to eat. Plus that volume expands our stomach, which signals our brain that we are full.

This means we can feel full even when eating far fewer calories.

Plus, processed foods are basically DESIGNED to cause us to want to keep eating. We get pleasure from eating those calorically dense, but nutritionally lacking foods.

And it is often much easier to eat those processed junk foods quickly. A candy bar can be gone in like a single bite!

Whole, natural foods often require you to slow down with your eating and take more bites, which helps prevent you from overeating partly because it allows your satiety signals to "keep up."

So while processed foods can have their place in a healthy, balanced diet, it is key we remember that whole, natural foods should be our main focus.

Not only are whole, natural foods important to our health, but they can also help us get better results faster!

What's "Clean?": Selecting A Dietary Preference

There are three parts to our diet we need to dial in based on our needs and goals.

-Macros
-Calories
-Dietary Preference

And just like there is no one size fits all macro ratio or calorie intake, there is no one size fits all dietary preference.

So what is a dietary preference?

A dietary preference provides you with guidelines about what foods are healthiest and what foods should be avoided.

It helps you dial in the quality and TYPES of foods that you eat.

For instance, Vegan, Vegetarian, Paleo, and Gluten-Free are all dietary preferences to name just a few options.

While we may have certain intolerances or allergies that make a dietary preference a necessity, there are lots of different ways of eating that can work for different people.

The key is using these dietary preferences to help us build a foundation of whole, natural foods that we enjoy eating and that help us feel good.

I make a distinction here between diet and dietary preference, calling Vegan or Vegetarian or Paleo a dietary preference, because you can truly use any of those and select different macro breakdowns to reach your goals.

Too often we confuse low carb and Paleo when really they don't have to go hand in hand. For more on Paleo approved foods, see the chart on page 186.

So if you have a dietary preference, or a list of foods you like to eat, you can consume those foods while still changing up your macros, and your calories, to match your lifestyle, activity level and goals as they evolve over time!

Veggie Eater Vs. Meat Eater

When working with clients to create the nutritional plan right for them, I only have one thing I'll push - and that is a focus on protein.

Whether you are a veggie eater or a meat eater, protein is key.

If you believe that consuming meat isn't ideal for your health and you prefer not to eat it, great.

If you believe that consuming meat is ideal for your health and you prefer to eat it, great.

Reviewing the latest research I believe that if you focus on whole, natural foods and avoid processed foods as much as possible, you can see great health benefits and results either way.

I believe that you can get enough protein, and all of the nutrients that you need, on either type of diet.

(For a list of studies, comparing the longevity of health conscious Vegans, Vegetarians and Omnivores, check the references section in your digital program.)

The biggest issue we run into is that people select a dietary preference, even take for instance Paleo, and then end up eating processed foods while technically adhering to the guidelines.

We get lazy and enact the least healthy version of the dietary preference we are choosing to follow.

For instance, being Vegetarian and eating chips, isn't going to get you results even though that's technically a food you can eat as a Vegetarian.

So while you may or may not believe in consuming meat, your focus still needs to be on whole, natural foods and hitting those macros!

And when you do select a specific dietary preference, you need to be aware of the potential deficiencies or challenges you may encounter when eliminating specific foods or food groups from your diet.

Vegetarians:

For anyone starting a Vegetarian diet, it is key you make a conscious effort to avoid being deficient in many of the nutrients we automatically get from eating meat and animal products, like Vitamin B12, Iron and even Calcium.

When you do transition, it can be good to plan out meals ahead of time to make sure you're getting all of the nutrients you need. Make sure to adjust slowly as a sudden change can affect your digestive system, changing your gut microbiome and causing bloating.

Getting enough protein is also a challenge for many new Vegetarians.

Not getting sufficient protein may cause you to take longer to recover from your workouts and hinder proper muscle repair. You may also feel more fatigued and suffer from some hair loss.

So while you may not be eating meat, you still need to consume adequate amounts of protein. This is even key to helping you maintain proper brain functioning and avoid brain fog!

Make sure to check out my Complementary Proteins Chart as well as the Vegetarian recipes and meal plans to help you increase your protein intake if you need ideas on page 184!

Vegans:

Because Vegans don't eat dairy or eggs, they may find they initially need to do more planning to make sure they hit their macro breakdowns and micronutrient needs.

Getting enough Vitamin D is a main concern, especially during winter months. And a deficiency in this vitamin often isn't noticed until it is too late.

It is important to realize that when you make the switch to a Vegan diet, you need to be conscious to find sources of Vitamin D right away as your Vitamin D stores are thought to only last about 2 months.

Another common vitamin deficiency seen in Vegans, besides Iron and even Zinc, is Vitamin B12. This nutrient is essential to proper functioning of our blood and nerve cells.

Being conscious of the symptoms of B12 deficiency is key, which include breathlessness, exhaustion, memory loss and tingling in the hands and feet.

While B12 is found in animal products, a deficiency can be easily prevented by eating B12 fortified foods or by taking a supplement.

The key is to be aware that this nutrient is essential so you can make sure your diet meets your needs.

A deficiency in Vitamin B12 would also negate the benefits of a Vegan diet in terms of reducing your risk of heart disease and stroke while putting you at risk for permanent nerve and brain damage.

Calcium is another nutrient Vegans are often deficient in. There are vegetables rich in calcium, like broccoli and kale, so you can 100% meet your needs, you must just be conscious of this risk. Plant-based calcium is also harder to absorb so even considering supplementation or fortified foods can help.

There is a 30% increased risk of fracture among Vegans, when compared to Vegetarians and Omnivores, so by simply tracking your food as a Vegan, you can ensure you're reaping the benefits of a Vegan diet without the risks!

Vegans still need to focus on protein to get better results, especially when it comes to body composition changes!

Omnivores:

While being an Omnivore makes it easier to hit your protein goals and allows you to take advantage of the nutrients available in animal products, you can still end up with deficiencies if you aren't conscious about your food choices!

Because not all animal proteins contain all vitamins and minerals nor the same types of fats.

If you want to consume more Zinc, you may opt for oysters over red meat, especially if you're trying to lower your saturated fat intake.

Or to make sure you aren't deficient in two very important minerals, iodine and selenium, you may increase your fish and seafood intake.

You may also want to be conscious of the omega-6 to omega-3 ratio you are consuming.

You'll need to find a balance between consuming proteins higher in omega-6s, such as dark meat chicken and skin, and those richer in omega-3s, such as mackerel or trout.

Also, as an Omnivore, you still need to make fruits and vegetables a main focus. They contain a variety of vitamins and minerals we need to stay balanced and healthy.

Vitamin C is one vitamin that is most easily consumed from plant sources. It is key to helping lower our risk for cardiovascular disease, cancer, Alzheimer's disease and cataracts.

To increase your Vitamin C intake, include fruits and vegetables such as bell peppers, leafy greens, broccoli and kiwi.

No matter what…

No matter what dietary preference you select, you should be using that as a guideline to help you dial in the QUALITY of your foods based on your needs and goals.

And by tracking your food, you can help yourself prevent any deficiencies so you can get the most out of your nutrition plan!

When It May Be Time To Eliminate!

While I firmly believe we need to avoid making foods "off limits" whenever possible, if you have an allergy or an intolerance, you may have no choice.

If eating a food makes you feel bad, you'll want to eliminate that food from your diet, even if that food isn't technically an unhealthy one.

You'd be surprised by the number of seemingly "healthy" foods out there that cause certain people to have digestion issues.

Like broccoli.

Broccoli is often touted as one of the best vegetables for you, but for some, it can cause pain and bloating.

Or avocados. Or even blackberries.

Yup. Avocados are a healthy fat source and berries are rich in antioxidants, but both may cause you to have digestive issues.

Now just because they MAY cause issues doesn't mean you need to eliminate them.

That would be cutting off your nose to spite your face.

It would be eliminating some very healthy food options for no reason.

But for some people, these high FODMAP foods may be the cause of their digestive issues.

And just because something is "healthy," doesn't mean it is right for us.

Just remember, if you don't suffer any gas, bloating or general gastrointestinal distress when consuming these foods, there is no reason for you to eliminate them!

However, if you have IBS or unexplained digestion issues, you may want to consider investigating which foods seem to cause it.

Now what are FODMAPs?

FODMAP is an acronym for Fermentable, Oligosaccharides, Disaccharides, Monosaccharides And (this is the A) Polyols.

Many foods that contain one of these, aren't necessarily unhealthy.

While yes, polyols are found in sugar alcohols, they are also found in avocados, blackberries and nectarines to name a few. And that is just a few of the "Ps" that may cause digestive issues.

(For a full list of foods high in FODMAPs, see my FODMAP food chart!)

If you find you are having digestive issues, trying an elimination diet to determine the culprit may be key. While we never want to make foods off limits if it isn't warranted, our diet should help us feel better, not gassy or bloated!

If you aren't sure of the cause of your digestive issues, make sure to consult your doctor to even run tests.

Once you know your intolerances, you can create food guidelines to help yourself reach your goals.

For a list of low and high FODMAP foods, check out my FODMAP food chart on page 187.

Now, What About Calories? How Many Calories Do You Really Need?

We often hear the phrase, "It's calories in vs. calories out."

If you want to lose weight, you need to eat fewer calories than you burn.

If you want to gain weight, you need to eat more calories than you burn.

However, how do we know what actually puts us in a deficit or a surplus!?

Because not only can our individual energy needs be different, but we've learned that a calorie isn't really just simply a calorie all things considered.

The thing is…many factors affect the calorie intake that is right for us and our goals.

The macro breakdown we use can affect how our body responds.

How much we fidget and are active throughout the day, not including our exercise, can impact things.

Our workouts, and even how we adapt to them over time, can affect things.

And of course, the metabolism you are born with, or the metabolic rate you now have because of your dieting practices, can change your caloric needs.

Age can also be a factor to consider.

While it doesn't have as much of an impact as we give it credit for, hormonal changes, and even our struggles to retain lean muscle mass, can affect things. Although often it is actually more of the LIFESTYLE CHANGES we make as we get older that affect our calorie burn.

The point is there are lots of things that can affect how many calories you really need and these needs can change day to day or even over the weeks or months as other lifestyle factors change and we move closer to our goals!

The key is figuring out a basic calorie range we can start with and adjusting from there.

I say a RANGE because I think too often, if we have one set specific number, we get very scared of even the slightest deviation from that number.

By giving yourself a range, even if just a small range of 100 calories plus or minus to start, you allow yourself to respond a bit more to hunger cues or slight changes in activity level. It also allows you to experiment and not stress over perfection in hitting a "cap."

Because the calorie intake we first start with is really just a GUIDE, especially when we've never hit certain macros or worked toward specific goals before.

And we shouldn't fear adjusting our calorie intake over time as our needs change.

If our lifestyle changes and we become less active? We may need fewer calories.

If we start lifting and building muscle? We may then need more calories.

If we lose weight? We may find we need fewer calories to maintain our new weight to start.

Then, over time, as we've sustained the weight loss for longer, we may find we end up needing to increase our calories.

Our metabolism does adapt and change.

The question is, with all of these factors to consider, where do you start?

I usually use a few very BASIC calorie calculations.

Ultimately, it's going to be about tracking and logging your food, and your progress, to adjust over time.

I even recommend, if you have no idea how many calories you are currently consuming, FIRST tracking your intake for a week.

This way you can make small adjustments to what you're currently doing.

Because if you are consuming far more calories than you calculate you "should" be consuming with the calculations below, you may end up feeling super hungry from instantly dropping them.

Instead, if you find you're eating far more, you can slowly, and incrementally, lower your intake over the weeks to avoid these feelings of hunger that often lead to us falling off of our diet.

By adjusting based on where you are currently, you may realize that you should have used a higher calculation to start OR you may end up getting down to that new number and achieving the results you want!

Same rules apply if you're eating far less than you calculate you "should" be. While, yes, a deficit is key if you want to lose weight, eating too little can hinder you from getting results.

Severe calorie deprivation inhibits the production of serotonin, a brain chemical needed to control appetite and curb cravings.

When we don't eat enough, we can make ourselves feel even hungrier than we actually are, which is what can lead to those cravings and binges you can't stop or control!

Eating in too extreme a deficit can also lead to weight gain because it can cause imbalanced hormone levels and your metabolism to down regulate as an adaptation to the lack of energy.

Your body will start to conserve energy if not enough fuel is coming in, which means you'll burn fewer calories throughout the day.

Because you're burning fewer calories, you'll need to consume less, which is why it can feel like you need to keep eating less and less to make any progress.

But if you do continue to lower your calories, it turns into a nasty cycle that often puts us right back where we started!

If you are undereating, slowly raising your calories may actually kickstart your weight loss. But again, you want to make small, incremental changes instead of dramatically changing your calorie intake, especially if you are also adjusting macro ratios at the same time.

Simple Calorie Calculations To Get You Started!

Kickstarting Weight Loss And Fat Loss:

Depending on your exact activity level, and how close you are to your goal, generally a calculation of between 10-12 x goal bodyweight is a good place to start.

Really looking for that kickstart and not that active?

If you're looking to lose weight, and even overcome a plateau, but not as active, I recommend using 10x goal bodyweight (in pounds).

This calculation works well if you are just starting back to light workouts a couple of times a week or not working out at all. It will help you see progress quickly to stay motivated and even get the ball rolling after being stuck at a plateau.

If you are more active but still looking for that kickstart to shed fat and lose weight?

While you may choose to still use 10x goal bodyweight for a 2 week kickstart, or to finish a cut, you may find that 11x goal bodyweight is more appropriate.

This calculation will still allow for fast results while keeping you more energized and is a great place to start for weight and fat loss, especially if you are active but have a desk job.

Super active and more focused on fat loss or even starting to transition into maintaining your results?

If you're nearing your goal and working out hard, maybe you just have those last few pounds of fat you want to lose, 12x goal bodyweight can be a great place to start.

When you have just that last little bit of fat to lose, you need to create a smaller deficit and even adjust macros. Results may happen slower, but you want to make sure you are just losing fat and not muscle.

If you have more weight to lose and aren't as active, but have tracked your food and are eating higher calorie, you may start with this calculation and then slowly increase your deficit instead of creating a more dramatic deficit to start.

More experienced long distance runners, with the goal of weight loss, may start with this calculation while upping their mileage before their peak training period.

Newbie runners, or those new to exercise in general, will find it easier to lose weight at the start because of the increase in activity so may need to keep their calories higher.

However, if you are a runner in your off season and your runs are more controlled, and because your body adapts more quickly to steady-state cardio, you may want to consider a few weeks of cycling down to 11x goal bodyweight.

Always On The Go? Looking To Continue To Improve Your Body Composition Or Maintain Your Results?

If you're always active and have a metabolism that others may curse you for, you're going to want to use a calorie calculation of 13-15x goal bodyweight. And your goal bodyweight may be what you're at currently or even higher. Our goals don't always have to be less!

This range is also a great place to start if you're looking to transition into a maintenance phase.

Basically…If you never seem to sit down, are always on the go, training hard, sometimes even training more than once a day, still wanting to lean down a bit or even wanting to gain muscle without putting on a ton of fat, this is where you should start.

Setting a range here is even more key as you really want to focus on fueling your training.
You'll want to start between 13-14x goal bodyweight.

This isn't necessarily day to day cycling, but more if you have an active day, or lift heavier that day, you may want to give yourself the freedom to respond to your hunger and fuel your activity.

Or if you have an unscheduled day off or simply aren't as hungry, you also want to have a range to respond to those cues while still fueling the rest of your week.

Often we stall our fat loss progress by training hard and NOT EATING ENOUGH!

And if gaining muscle is your primary goal, you need to eat even more!

You may even find, especially depending on your ratio, that you need 15x goal bodyweight (in lbs). Hardgainers really dedicated to a bulk may even adjust up to 16-17x goal bodyweight.

Remember, if you want to gain, a surplus is key!

You do not want to feel hungry during this phase of your diet, but you also want to track things for as clean a bulk as possible if you don't want to put on a ton of extra fat as you gain muscle!

Getting Started Using These Calculations:

Using these simple calculations, you can start to create a calorie range for yourself based on your basic activity level and goals.

You will then use this number, or range, to calculate your macros based on the ratio you select. I'll be going over ratios based on a variety of goals and needs.

The key, once you have a starting calorie intake, is to track, tweaking those basic ranges to tailor them to meet YOUR SPECIFIC NEEDS!

Remember, there are so many factors that make our needs unique, even including how we've dieted in the past!

Why You May Need To Start Lower And ADD Calories:

Eating too little can hinder your results just as badly as eating too much.

Often, and I see it most often with my female clients, we cut calories too low in an attempt to lose fat faster. We do this even as we increase our training intensity in an attempt to burn more calories.

So not only are we cutting our energy intake, but we're, at the same time, trying to increase our calorie expenditure.

Doing both things at once most often backfires, leading to health issues (including missed periods or no periods for women) and even weight gain...the exact opposite of what we were hoping to accomplish.

It can make us feel like we've damaged our metabolism.

We're eating less yet our weight isn't changing because our metabolism slows in response to the reduced energy consumption.

However, this "damage" isn't permanent.

It's merely an adaption we can reverse. It's our body's way of protecting itself.

To start to "heal" our metabolism, and even kickstart our results again, we often need to simply eat more.

But this doesn't mean you should just start going crazy with the calories.

You need to make this adjustment SLOWLY. You almost have to train your body to eat more.

So if you've been in a deficit for maybe too long and have plateaued, slowly start increasing your calories each week or two.

You may even continue with the macro ratio you were using, or slightly increase protein, as you up your calories. This can help you avoid gaining extra fat.

We have to remember that our dieting practices in the past can really influence our current needs.

Bumping calories too quickly can lead us back into a yo-yo dieting cycle because we just end up gaining back the fat we lost.

We have to retrain our body because it has been taught by us to conserve.

We want to use the slow calorie increase to help fuel our workouts so we can build muscle, and strengthen our metabolism.

Remember when we put our body in an extreme deficit, it will catabolize even our muscle tissue for energy. And less muscle means fewer calories burned while at rest (aka a slower metabolism).

This is another reason to give yourself a calorie range to work in to start and not be afraid to adjust over time, responding to your hunger cues even as you track.

It's also why you have to remember it isn't simply calories in vs calories out. More of a deficit or more of a surplus isn't always better.

Plus often a plateau doesn't have to mean just adjusting calories. You sometimes simply need a change in your macro breakdown to kickstart your results! Specifically, don't always turn to cutting out more calories!

Don't be hesitant to set a range but LISTEN TO YOUR BODY especially as you learn what your true hunger signals are!

Creating Your Diet Plan

Now comes the fun part, determining the ratios right for you so you can get started eating according to your goals!

But first, it's key you understand what those macro ratios listed with each goal really mean.

While using a fitness tracker is the easiest way to use the ratios, as then all of the math is done for you, it is never bad to understand how you can do the math on your own.

I recommend calculating a caloric intake for yourself right now so you can try the math yourself with the ratio I use in the following example!

What Do Those Macro % Really Mean?

Often, and especially in this program, you will see macro breakdowns listed as percentages.

Those percentages represent the amount of your daily calorie intake that should come from each macro.

So if your ratio says 40% protein, 30% carbs, 30% fat, that means 40% of your calories should come from protein, 30% from carbs and 30% from fat.

If you use a food tracker, you'll notice that these percentages change over the course of a day. You can see these percents in the pie chart most fitness trackers provide.

This is because, as we log our meals, the charts show the percentage of our current calories consumed that come from each macronutrient.

What you want to focus on is not the changes after each meal, BUT instead hitting the ratio at the end of the day when you've consumed your desired calorie intake.

So when you've hit your calorie intake at the end of the day, the pie chart should THEN show the ratio you've chosen to follow.

After one meal, if your ratio is at 50% carbs, just remember that the chart is showing you the breakdown of that specific meal.

You haven't gone over your carb allotment for the day!

To find out how much protein, carbs and fat you need for the entire day, I recommend using the ratio you've selected, and your calorie intake, to calculate the GRAMS of each macro you should be consuming in total.

This way, even as the chart percentages change, you will know how much of each macronutrient you have left.

While many trackers will show you the total grams you need to consume based on the macro ratios entered, in MyFitnessPal it's under the Nutrients tab next to the Macro tab with the pie chart, you can also do the calculations yourself.

EXAMPLE:

Let's say your calorie intake is 1,500. Take your calorie intake and multiple it by the percent of each macro you plan to consume.

Using the 40% protcin, 30% carb, 30% fat ratio I mentioned above...

40% protein x 1500 calories = 600 calories from protein
30% carbs x 1500 calories = 450 calories from carbs
30% fat x 1500 calories = 450 calories from fat

Next you'll divide the calories you calculated above for each macro by the calories per gram of each macronutrient.

-Protein has 4 calories per gram
-Carbs have 4 calories per gram
-Fat has 9 calories per gram

So...

600 calories of protein per day/4 calories per gram = 150 grams of protein
450 calories of carbs per day/4 calories per gram = 112.5 grams of carbs
450 calories of fat per day/9 calories per gram = 50 grams of fat

These are the total grams of each macronutrient you need to eat per day if you want to hit a macro ratio of

40% protein, 30% carbs and 30% fat at 1,500 calories.

So once you've selected your ratio, and calculated your calories, you can calculate how many grams of each macro you need.

The nice thing about a food tracker app is it does all of this for you!

And, after you've selected your ratio and calculated your calories, you can even use one of the meal plans I've included in this book to help you get started if you aren't sure how to hit those totals!

Planning ahead is also key as you learn to hit those totals. Even try mapping out some of your own meal prep ideas!

And if you aren't sure what foods are made up of what macros, check my Macro Cheat Sheet to help you get started on page 183!

Creating Your Plan Is One Big Experiment!

I think it is human nature to always want to improve - to constantly seek out and try new things in an attempt to get better/stronger/faster/leaner...

It's why, when we've reached a goal, say we've lost the weight we wanted to lose, we will instantly set another one.

Maybe we'll work to get a flatter stomach. Or put on some muscle. Or fuel a race we plan to train for.

We are constantly testing and tweaking and adapting our routines, our diets, to help us get better and better results and reach new goals.

Everything is an experiment!

And that is why it is so key we track our nutrition to see how it affects our progress.

You can't change and tweak what you are doing if you don't have an accurate picture of the actions you've taken.

You won't know if you're more fat-adapted, carb-adapted or metabolically flexible unless you test out different ratios based on your goals.

And with each goal, I'll help you match your ratios to your needs with options no matter what macros you run best on!

The key is setting a plan and sticking to it as you track your progress toward your goal.

Even when you get the results you want, and your plan seems amazing, at some point those results may slow no matter how amazing your plan is.

Sometimes your body simply needs a change.

Making adjustments doesn't mean that what you were doing was bad or wrong.

Remember, our bodies do adapt and change over time!

So if you're progress slows, if you get bored, if your lifestyle or goals change, don't be afraid to adapt and adjust.

But make sure you first actually give yourself time to see what works and what doesn't.

This is why I recommend cycling ratios every 1-6 weeks.

Cycling Your Ratios

If you aren't hitting the ratios you set, you don't know if those ratios will work.

The first rule with macro cycling is that you have to consistently hit your breakdown BEFORE you think about switching to a new breakdown.

When you're first starting out, this may mean spending an extra week dialing in your ratios.

It is also why planning ahead, if you're new to tracking macros, can be key so that you can hit your ratios that very first day you start!

And with each macro breakdown, you may stay on a ratio for anywhere between 1-6 weeks.

I don't recommend cycling your ratios daily as it is not necessary for most of us and far more complicated. And it can lead to worse results if you aren't very meticulous in your tracking!

The only time this daily cycling may really pay off is if you're looking to reach that extra level of leanness for a specific event or competition and you've stalled trying everything else. I will touch on this in the Six Pack Macros section.

Otherwise you will stick with the same ratio for a full week or even up to 6 weeks straight.

Adjusting Your Ratios Weekly:

If you're more experienced with logging, and really looking to kickstart or accelerate your results, alternating ratios every week works well.

If you're also training for a specific race or competition, you may adjust your ratios every week leading up to the competition as your training peaks.

Adjusting Your Ratios Every 2-4 Weeks:

If you're goal is weight loss or fat loss, switching things up every 2-4 weeks can help you avoid plateaus while also getting into a routine with your diet.

This allows you to keep a consistent energy source to fuel your training as well, which can be key to getting fat loss and weight loss results more quickly.

You may even find you time the adjustments to your macros with changes in your workout programming. This works really well if you cycle and create new workouts every 2-4 weeks when you change your ratio.

Even when maintaining your weight or looking to add muscle, you may find switching things up at this frequency allows you to keep your meal prep interesting without creating more stress.

However, the more you're focused on building, the more consistent you will want to be with your fuel so the less frequently you will want to adjust.

Also, when starting prep for a race or competition, you will want to stay with ratios for longer as your focus should be on your training.

Adjusting Your Ratios Every 4-6 Weeks:

Even if you're simply maintaining, every so often, you'll want to change things up!

Our brains also do well with an END DATE…even when it's a lifestyle.

So adjusting ratios, even if you're not looking to achieve any specific goal, can help you prevent backsliding and potentially even help you find something you enjoy more.

It's not uncommon to feel like you've stalled around that 5-6 week mark.

Adjusting our diet, even if we haven't stalled, can also help provide us with some variety to our meals as we often find new recipes to match our new breakdowns.

Whether you're looking to maintain, add muscle or focus on fueling your training, you may find sticking with your breakdown for a bit longer works well.

But even then, we do want to cycle!

Select Your Macro Breakdown Based On Your Goals

Whether we want to lose weight, fuel our race training or gain muscle, there are different macro ratios we can use to eat according to our goals.

And in the next sections, I'll share with you the tips, "tricks," and macros you need to get results for all of those different goals. While I recommend reading through all of the sections at some point, you can start by skipping to the section that matches your needs so you can get started today.

But first, you need to answer this question for yourself…"What is your main goal?"

You may want to lose weight AND gain muscle AND train for a race, but you want to have one goal be your main focus to start.

And your goal can even be that you're just starting out and simply want to make the switch to a healthier overall lifestyle. (If this is your goal, the Beginner's Macro section is the perfect place to start!)

Once you know your main goal, you can skip to that section:

-Beginner's Macros
-Weight Loss Macros
-Six Pack Macros (Fat Loss Macros)
-Muscle Macros
-Maintenance Macros
-Endurance Sport Macros
-Managing Hormones

And ladies, I recommend reading not only the section about your goal, but also the "Managing Hormones" section to help you navigate those different hormonal changes as you work toward your specific goals. In this section, I'll discuss eating not only around your period but even menopause!

For each goal I've included, you'll find not only the macro ratios and ranges you need to get results but also some amazing recipes and meal plans to help you get started.

I even go over cheat days or refeed days, supplements and all of those other little tweaks we can make to tailor our diet to meet our specific needs and lifestyles.

Time to get started eating according to your goals to get the lean, strong body you've always wanted!

Beginner's Macros

When you're just getting started, especially if you've never tracked macros before, it can all feel a bit overwhelming and intimidating.

It can feel like there are just so many changes to make and that you need to make them all at once.

But that isn't the case! Let's start by breaking down the changes into manageable pieces!

Where Do You Start?

If change seems intimidating, your first move should be to simply figure out what you are currently doing.

Just start tracking, which I've mentioned before.

Enter the calories you want to hit and the ratios you plan to use and then just simply track.

Don't try to change anything. Don't cut out any foods.

Just log.

Often just the accountability of tracking, just seeing what you are truly doing, gets you to start tweaking and making changes.

They may be small changes, and often it's simply that we skip that extra snack or make an effort to get more veggies, but we start to make changes and that is what matters.

Those changes alone will add up.

After you log for just a week without judgment, seeing how close you really are to your macro and calorie goals, you can then start making changes. And the bonus is, tracking will have already become a habit!

Start With Something Easy:

As you log make note of what you seem to struggle with the most.

Make note of things you seem to "need" or crave and also the things that don't really matter as much that may be easier to cut out.

All too often, we first try to cut out those things we crave and enjoy the most.

But instead, find things you can tweak that AREN'T as important to you.

Find one thing you can change that almost seems too easy to swap out or adjust.

Add in one more ounce of protein. Cut out those few crackers you snack on.

Swap that sugar-packed processed cereal for a homemade oatmeal dish with protein.

Add in veggies to your usual pasta.

Make a simple swap that moves you closer to your ultimate goal.

Start with something easy to change because, being able to make that change quickly and easily, will only motivate you to continue to move forward. It lowers your defenses against making further changes!

Commit To One Change:

After you start logging, commit to focusing on ONE change.

This focus on one thing can help you continue to move forward and see big progress without becoming overwhelmed.

Because of the importance of protein to our weight loss, muscle gaining and performance goals, I always recommend starting there.

Most often too, our protein intake is below where we want it to be. So focus first on just increasing protein.

Don't worry about where your carbs or fat fall to start. And don't worry about cutting out the foods you love.

Just tweak recipes and meals to hit your protein intake.

While you may want to adjust the overall quality of the foods you eat, first just focus on hitting your macros. You may be surprised by how much just focusing on those macros can help you make other changes, like eating more whole natural foods.

Also, small swaps toward more quality foods adds up.

Maybe you'd like to ideally eat chicken and veggies for a meal but are currently eating processed pizza. First start with making yourself a macro-friendly pizza, maybe even with some chicken and veggies on it or a salad on the side.

It's healthier and will help you hit your macros so you can see results. Those results will keep you motivated so you can keep building toward what you'd ideally like to do.

And even though the macro-friendly pizza may still be slightly processed, it helps you start to get CONSISTENT and moving forward.

Plus, it's still better nutritionally than what you were doing. Being "better" is more important than being "perfect." Because "better" allows for us to build lasting habits.

The key is to commit to changing ONE THING FIRST and allow that change to direct and guide other changes.

Don't Expect Perfection:

No one, even someone who has been following a healthy lifestyle for years, is going to be perfect every day. And perfection isn't required for results.

Consistency is!

So as you make changes, don't feel like a day is ruined if it isn't perfect.

Just focus on moving forward, knowing that deviations from our plan will happen.

Life is going to get in the way and we just have to work around it.

If you have an "off day," a day you wish you could "do over"...well...the simple fact is...you can't.

All you can do is learn from it and move forward. Maybe you can reflect and find a way to plan better in the future.

Or maybe you just chalk it up to unforeseen circumstances and keep moving forward, making your next meal one that is back on track.

Don't make yourself feel guilty. And especially don't get down if you're just a few percents off the ratios.

Ratios are GUIDES. As you start out, if you get within 2-3% of your goal, you should consider that an amazing victory and essentially perfection.

Dietary preferences are also just guides.

For example, if you don't have a gluten intolerance and indulge in bread, even though it's not "Paleo approved," don't stress or worry. Log it, focus on hitting your ratios and move forward!

The key is consistency and constantly working to find better and better ways to work toward our goals!

PLAN PLAN PLAN:

You need to plan ahead when you first start because often our habits are nowhere near close to what they need to be.

We've probably even created some super unhealthy habits that are so "natural" we don't even realize we do them.

By planning ahead, we give ourselves a guide to avoid those old and unhealthy habits.

We can make sure we have meals prepped and ready for those busy days when we might otherwise reach for something that won't help us reach our goals.

We can even use planning ahead to help us when we have to eat out.

A dinner out with friends?

Check out the menu ahead of time and plan the rest of your day around it. Even if you don't know the exact macros of the meal, you can guestimate close enough and give yourself more wiggle room for that meal out by eating lower calorie and higher protein earlier in the day.

Planning ahead can even allow you to map in some restaurant dishes for when you travel or for those days you might not be able to meal prep.

Planning ahead helps make things less overwhelming by showing us what we need to do to hit our calories and macros. It can help us create those new habits that make eating according to our goals more intuitive.

And when you plan ahead, keep things simple.

There is nothing wrong with wanting to eat a variety of foods. But when you first start out, picking a few meals, a few ingredients, to focus on can help.

Too often we try to get too fancy with our prep, which only makes logging and hitting our macros harder.

And if, starting out, you feel overwhelmed by the idea of planning your own meals from scratch, check out one of the meal plans I've included for beginners. These can help you get moving forward without the hassle of figuring anything out to start.

And by logging these days as you start out, you can give yourself a base off of which to build future meal plans!

While you may want to learn how to meal plan for yourself, sometimes having someone else map out a plan for you first can be key and help give you ideas. It can make the initial changes easier since you don't have to figure out how to hit the ratios yourself.

It's also why you can find out more about getting your own custom map in your Macro Hacks digital edition or by going to the link below!

redefiningstrength.com/hacks

But before you start, review the recipes and meal plans I've included so you can see and understand portion sizes and recipes that could work for you!

Don't Go It Alone:

The ups and downs - the victories and the setbacks - that come with making changes can be amazing, but also hard.

It's why having a support group, or making changes with a spouse or friend can make things easier!

Not only can they provide support and accountability, but they can also make the whole process more fun!

Do the planning and prepping together. Get your family cooking and involved.

Online communities can also work well for accountability and even for ideas and recipes. You can even see how others have made the changes.

That's why it's also important you join the private Redefining Strength Facebook (find the link to access the group in your digital edition).

You'll then have the support of others who've also made the change to tracking macros!

And it is a perfect place to share your struggles and celebrate your victories.

No one has ever had success without failure. No one's journey is free from setbacks.

And having a community to support you through your ups and downs so you can keep moving forward, is so key!

Knowing you are not alone really helps!

So...What Ratios Are Best For Beginners?

As a beginner, you may want to first focus on logging, then add or subtract grams of each macro from there.

A great way to get started, if you're struggling with the idea of planning to hit a set ratio, is to make changes based on where you are at currently.

Take your current macros and enter the calorie intake you plan to hit.

If weight loss is your goal, 10-12x goal bodyweight is a good place to start.

If you have more than 70+ pounds to lose, or even just more than 30 pounds, you may want to start with a "goal bodyweight" that isn't your ultimate goal weight. This will help you avoid creating a massive calorie deficit to start.

Once you have your calorie goal, start by adjusting ONE MACRO by just 3-5% that week.

The macro that we most often need to increase is protein. So I recommend starting there. It is easier to focus on the macro you need to ADD to, over trying to subtract from somewhere else.

Find just one little tweak you can make to move yourself forward toward your goals. When you've mastered that 3-5% increase, make another adjustment until you hit the macro ratio you planned to start with.

What macro ranges should you start with?

Protein: Beginners should shoot for a protein intake between 25-40% of their total calories. While ideally for weight loss, you'll want 30-40% of your calories coming from protein, even just 25% to start may seem like a lot.

Carbs: For carbs, you can shoot for a range between 20-50%. While a wide range, this will come down to what you feel best with and even where your current carb intake is. The standard American diet ratio is 50% carbs so you may find it easier to start with a higher carb intake. And if you're also starting more intense exercise as you change your diet, especially endurance activities, the extra carbs may be helpful to stay energized. But even if you start with a higher carb ratio, it isn't bad to cycle through a lower carb ratio to test out how you react!

Fat: Fat intake will vary as much as carb intake, ranging from 20-50% of your calories coming from fat. If your current diet is higher in fat and lower in carbs, start with a ratio that allows you to maintain that high fat intake. You can then cycle and test out a lower fat ratio later. If you are also just starting out, and less active, a lower carb and higher fat ratio may work best.

What ratios can you use?

For beginners, these are 5 great specific breakdowns to use and cycle:

-35% protein/33% carb/32% fat (or fat and carbs about even)
-30% protein/50% carbs/20% fat
-30% protein/30% carbs/40% fat
-30% protein/20% carbs/50% fat
-40% protein/30% carbs/30% fat

All of these ratios are higher protein. For many beginners, keeping all of the macros about even is a good place to start.

Whether you find you are consuming more carbs or more fat, you will want to start with a ratio as close as possible to what you are currently doing to make the change easier.

How should you cycle the ratios?

While you will want to cycle the ratios, just remember that you must first actually HIT the numbers before you consider making changes.

I recommend staying with a ratio for 3-4 weeks as you get the hang of things. Even 5-6 weeks can work as long as you're continuing to see progress and making changes to your workout routine.

Below are 3 different cycling options for beginners looking to lose weight.

They are 9 week cycles, but you can extend them out to 12 weeks.

Cycle #1 is moderate ratios.

Cycle #2 is low carb ratios.

And Cycle #3 is experimental ratios.

Cycle #1 - Moderate:

A great beginner weight loss cycle, these ratios work well if you first need to focus on increasing protein and aren't sure if higher or lower carb works better for you. This is also a great cycle for those that are metabolically flexible aka they run equally well off of carbs and fat.

These ratios can be a good place to start too if your logs aren't leaning one way or the other in terms of high carb or high fat. (Many of these ratios, by adapting your calories, can also be a great way for you to maintain your results later on!)

Weeks 1-3: 35% protein/33% carbs/32% fat
Weeks 4-6: 30% protein/30% carbs/40% fat
Weeks 7-9: 40% protein/30% carbs/30% fat

Cycle #2 - Low Carb:

Especially if you have more weight to lose, and may not be working out or very active, lower carb ratios can help you get faster results to start. You simply don't need the easily available energy that carbs offer plus the higher fat ratios can keep you feeling fuller.

By cycling down in fat over the weeks while increasing protein, we can take advantage of the thermic effect of protein since, the more overweight we are, the less we benefit from any thermic effect that fat can have.

Carbs also increase over the weeks as generally our activity level increases during our weight loss journey.

Weeks 1-3: 30% protein/20% carbs/50% fat
Weeks 4-6: 30% protein/30% carbs/40% fat
Weeks 7-9: 40% protein/30% carbs/30% fat

Cycle #3 - Experimental:

If you aren't sure whether you feel better on higher or lower carb, and may even currently be consuming more carbs, this 9 week cycle is a great place to start. It will allow you to test out both a higher carb and higher fat ratio to see how you feel on each.

The moderate cycle in between will make for an easier transition between the two while still helping you move forward on your weight loss journey!

Weeks 1-3: 30% protein/50% carbs/20% fat
Weeks 4-6: 35% protein/33% carbs/32% fat
Weeks 7-9: 30% protein/20% carbs/50% fat

While you can create your own cycle using not only the breakdowns, but ranges I've included, these three options are a great place to start if you aren't sure how best to combine them.

And each of these ratios has a great meal plan with recipes you can check out to help you get started!

Should You Include Cheat Days, Macro Cheat Days Or Diet Breaks?

You don't want to deprive yourself when you're first starting out. Because the second you say something is off limits, you want it even more.

So while you can eat anything technically on any day, we all have those foods that trigger further cravings.

We all have those treats that we can't have just one of and stop.

And for those treats and indulgences, it can be key to save them for a day that we don't have to be as moderate on.

If you find there are foods you struggle to completely cut out, BUT that you can't indulge in moderately, it may be key to include a "Cheat Day" in your plan.

It's okay to want to have a day where you indulge in foods that you know aren't as healthy for you, even including alcohol. For the fastest results possible, keep alcohol to your cheat day, or completely eliminate it, especially when first starting out.

Cheat days can provide the mental break we need to stay consistent long term just make sure they don't lead to feelings of guilt!

If you have parties or meals out, where you know you won't be able to stay on track, plan those in as Cheat Days or even simply Cheat Meals. This allows you the freedom to indulge without feeling guilty.

However, if you've just started tracking, and have more weight to lose, it is best to skip a Cheat Day, or bigger calorie spike day, for the first 2-3 weeks. You want that calorie deficit to add up.

We have to remember that a day with a huge calorie spike can throw us out of a deficit for the week, even if we ate in a deficit potentially every other day.

So beginners should avoid a Cheat Day until they are 2-3 weeks into their plan.

If you also find indulging without limits sets off a bad cycle of binging, you may find a "Macro Cheat Day" works better for you.

On these days, you can set either a calorie limit to stay under or a macro ratio you still want to hit.

But either way, you'll provide yourself with a guide while spiking your calories slightly. A spike of 500-1000 calories can be acceptable, depending on how frequently you include these days and how long you've been dieting for.

These days become more beneficial the longer you've been in a calorie deficit. They help prevent unnecessary metabolic adaptation aka they can help keep your metabolism "healthy."

So as you move through even one of the 9 week cycles I created, you may want to include some form of a Macro Cheat Day or Cheat Day to spike your calories depending on which works best for you!

In terms of a dieting break, this will come into play as you get a bit closer to your goals. To use a dieting break, you'll take a 7-14 day "break" from your diet while eating at maintenance calories.

While this can slow down results, it can be a good way to shed that last bit of fat without losing muscle.

When you're just starting out, it is better to go less aggressive with your deficit, and maintain that one calorie intake, over cycling between a more aggressive deficit and "maintenance" calories like you would with a dieting break.

So don't worry about diet breaks until you start to focus more on fat loss and losing those last few pounds!

Supplements For Beginners

Supplements are supplemental.

They make the most difference the closer we are to our goals and the more we need those final little "tweaks."

The only supplements I recommend for someone starting out are protein powder and collagen, especially if your initial protein intake is low.

And I recommend them for beginners mainly because they can make things easier. And easier changes are not only...well...easier to make, but also easier to stick to!

Protein powders and shakes make for easy grab and go snacks. Protein powders and collagen can also be added to some of our favorite snack recipes to easily boost our protein intake.

Dessert recipes that also use protein powder can help us satisfy our sweet tooth while still staying on track as well!

They can also be an easy way for anyone who is Vegetarian or Vegan to increase their protein intake as they learn other ways to meal plan and prep.

So don't get bogged down looking at the supplements out there. Keep things simple.

Focus first on those macros and calories and getting those fundamentals in line. Once the basics are dialed in, and you've started making progress toward your goals, then you can consider playing around with supplements.

Weight Loss Macros

Weight loss is often the reason we really start paying attention to what we're eating - to our diet.

And while our goal may be to see a specific number on the scale, what we really want is to look leaner and more toned.

So even though weight loss may be your goal, you want to focus on retaining as much lean muscle mass as you can as you shed body fat.

This will even help you get better results faster.

While with weight loss we will lose some muscle mass, we want to prevent as much loss as possible by focusing on our macros over trying to create a more extreme calorie deficit.

Where Do You Start?

You may find you've lost weight in the past by simply cutting out certain foods, by going Paleo or Gluten-Free or becoming a Vegetarian.

Because by eliminating foods, we often end up lowering our calorie intake. Depending on the diet even, we automatically increase our protein too.

But to keep the momentum going, to get not only continued results but better and lasting results, we need to dial in our macro ratios and know what we are truly consuming.

Because not only are proper macro ratios key to helping us improve our body composition as we lose weight, but they can also help us understand why results may have stalled and what to do to keep moving forward.

Knowing the breakdown of your food can help you avoid having to restrict certain foods forever if you don't want to!

Also, by focusing on macro ratios and the calorie deficit you create, you can avoid feeling like you're constantly just having to cut out more and more to get results!

Remember going to low with your calories can hinder your weight loss, and especially fat loss, results!

Creating A Deficit

Most people set their calorie deficit without thought as to how their macros may affect it.

The thing is, your macro ratios can really affect the number of calories you feel you need and even the deficit that you're actually creating.

Because protein has a higher thermic effect, you may end up eating more calories than you "think" you should while still ending up in a deficit.

And when creating a calorie deficit, it's key you also don't drop your calories too low, too fast.

Our bodies, and especially our minds, DO NOT like change.

So creating less of a deficit can be helpful to start as we won't feel as hungry.

And often, simply by adjusting our macros while staying at our current calorie intake, we can begin to see weight loss results.

However, if you know you won't stick to your plan if you don't see fast results, you may want to start with a two week kickstart ratio and calorie intake aka something a bit more "aggressive" while having an exit strategy.

While those "fast" results are mainly due to water weight being lost and glycogen stores being depleted, they can still be motivating.

Just remember, we can only lose so much fat, without also losing muscle, in a single week.

So cutting our calories lower to try to lose faster on the scale could just result in more muscle mass being lost and a lower metabolic output.

What Calorie Calculation Should You Start With To Lose Weight?

If you have a desk job and aren't working out consistently or intensely, start with just 10x goal bodyweight.

If you are training consistently, 2-3 times a week, but not very active outside of those sessions, you may even find that 10x goal bodyweight works for you, especially as a kickstart.

If you use this lower ratio and are hungry after 4 days of dialing your macros, you may decide to up your calorie intake. But give yourself a few days to adjust to the change, especially if the macro ratios are dramatically different from what you were doing.

This calculation is a great way to create a slightly more aggressive deficit and build momentum to get the ball rolling.

But you want to be conscious not to stay in too big a deficit for too long as you don't want to lose muscle or cause yourself to binge eat.

And when you use that 10x goal bodyweight calculation, you may use your FIRST goal weight, not your ultimate goal weight.

If you have more than 30+ pounds to lose, you may want to set an initial goal weight less than halfway to your ultimate goal weight, then adjust from there.

You want to avoid decreasing calories by much more than 500 below what you are currently doing. So you may want to use a calculation more between 11-12, or even 13, x goal bodyweight.

For those of us working out consistently, and even intensely, staying between 11-12x goal bodyweight may work best. You want to fuel your activity so you can retain lean muscle mass and actually get results faster.

If you are training hard and looking to lose those last few pounds, you may not only want to check out the

Six Pack Macros section, but even potentially stay between 12-14 x goal bodyweight (even setting your goal bodyweight as your current weight).

What Ratios Work Best?

Focusing on protein is key if you want to lose weight while avoiding losing muscle mass.

A high protein diet may even help you GAIN muscle while in a deficit.

So as you start tracking macros, first focus on hitting your protein intake, while not worrying about your exact carb or fat percentages.

Eating enough to protect your lean muscle can help prevent extreme metabolic adaptation.

You can keep your metabolic rate higher and burn more calories at rest the more muscle mass you have!

So what macro ranges should you use?

Protein: To lose weight and help yourself not only retain, but even gain muscle while in a deficit, keep your protein intake between 30-45%. You may think that you don't need as much protein if you aren't working out intensely, but that is not the case! The thermic effect of protein alone makes it a beneficial macro for weight loss. And especially if you're doing more steady state cardio, higher protein can help you avoid muscle catabolism. So focus first on protein!

Carbs: Your carb intake should be between 20-40% of your daily calorie intake. Especially if you are more active, competing in an endurance sport, or just have those last few pounds to lose, you may want to stay toward the upper end of that range. While if you are just starting your weight loss journey, and less active, you may want to go lower toward the end of that carb range. (If you are training for a race, even while trying to lose weight, make sure to check the Endurance Sport Macros.)

Fat: Keeping fat intake between 25-40% is a great way to make sure you feel full and fueled. The less active you are, or the more you need to see fast results to stay motivated, the higher you'll want to keep your fat intake while cutting carbs. If you do have only those last few pounds to lose, you may want to drop fat down to between 20-30%. For more fat loss ranges check the Six Pack or Fat Loss Macros section.

What ratios can you use?

For weight loss, these are 5 great specific breakdowns to use and cycle:

-30% protein/40% carbs/30% fat
-30% protein/30% carbs/40% fat
-30% protein/20% carbs/50% fat
-40% protein/30% carbs/30% fat
-45% protein/20% carbs/35% fat

These ratios are all high protein and tend toward higher fat, although you'll see that first ratio is carb focused. But going slightly lower carb to start can provide that bonus kickstart!

I mentioned you can lower fat to even 20-25% although I find this fat range more beneficial as your focus shifts more toward fat loss.

If you do want to drop fat a bit lower because you are active in endurance activities, consider these ranges:

-Protein: 35-40%
-Carbs: 35-40%
-Fat: 20-25%.

How should you cycle ratios?

While you will want to cycle ratios, just remember that you must first actually HIT the numbers before you consider making changes. You may find that the very first ratio you use takes you longer to adjust to than future cycles. So you may spend an extra week on that first breakdown but shorten the time spent on future ratios.

For weight loss, you'll want to cycle every 2-3 weeks. This keeps your results progressing and helps you avoid plateauing without lowering your calorie intake.

You may find, over the course of your weight loss journey, that you DO need to decrease calories as your energy expenditure changes. If you do, make sure to do so slowly and only if a simple adjustment to your macros doesn't do the trick first!

Below are 3 different cycling options.

They are all 6 week cycles, although you can extend them out to 9 weeks.

Cycle #1 is for those less active or who may not be working out at all.
Cycle #2 is for those returning to exercise or increasing their current activity level.

And Cycle #3 is for those working out intensely.

Cycle #1 - Not As Active:

If you aren't currently working out, or if you are training less frequently at a lower intensity, these ratios and 6 week cycle are the perfect place to start.

You'll start with a slightly more moderate ratio, which, while still high protein, is often an easier one to hit starting out. You'll then drop your carbs to speed up results slightly before bumping your carbs back up as you focus on increasing protein further. This will help you preserve lean muscle mass while keeping your hormones balanced.

Weeks 1-2: 30% protein/30% carbs/40% fat
Weeks 3-4: 30% protein/20% carbs/50% fat
Weeks 5-6: 40% protein/30% carbs/30% fat

Cycle #2 - Returning To Exercise/Increasing Activity:

While weight loss may be your primary goal, you want to also make sure you're fueling your workouts properly!

If we cut our calories too low or don't consume the proper macros, our workouts, can suffer.

And being able to increase our training intensity will only help us get results faster. So as you increase your activity level, your diet also has to adjust.

That's why you'll start out with slightly higher protein to help you build muscle even while in a deficit.

Then as you begin to adapt to your new exercise routine, you'll lower protein and even carbs. In the final weeks, you'll get a bit of a kickstart increasing protein while dropping carbs lower. Because you'll have adapted to the change in exercise, carbs won't be as necessary for instant fuel. These ratios will protect the lean muscle mass you've built while helping you continue to lose weight.

Weeks 1-2: 40% protein/30% carbs/30% fat
Weeks 3-4: 30% protein/30% carbs/40% fat
Weeks 5-6: 45% protein/20% carbs/35% fat

Cycle #3 - Training Hard:

If you're training intensely, make sure to also use one of those higher calorie calculations along with the ratios below.

To help you maintain your training intensity, the first ratio keeps your carb intake higher while still being high protein. This will help you avoid losing muscle while training intensely in a calorie deficit.

You'll then cycle up in protein over the weeks, to help you retain and even build muscle while in a deficit. And you will slowly lower carbs, to help you blast past any plateaus.

Do not be afraid to also increase calories over the weeks as you focus more on protein!

Weeks 1-2: 30% protein/40% carbs/30% fat
Weeks 3-4: 40% protein/30% carbs/30% fat
Weeks 5-6: 45% protein/20% carbs/35% fat

While you can create your own cycle using not only the breakdowns, but also the ranges I've included, these three options are a great place to start. And each of these ratios has a meal plan with recipes you can check out to help you get started!

Should You Include Cheat Days, Macro Cheat Days Or Diet Breaks?

Depending on where you're at in your weight loss journey, all of these things can be used to help you get consistent and stay on track long term.

They can even help you create that elusive "lifestyle" once you've reached your weight loss goal!

With weight loss, it is all about consistency.

And Cheat Days, Macro Cheat Days and even Dieting Breaks can all help you stay consistent. The key is using the ones that are best for YOU personally because any can work if they also fit with your lifestyle and mindset.

Cheat Days, or even Cheat Meals, are more free-for-alls. We don't care or have any limits. We simply eat what we want.

Macro Cheat Days are days we can still eat anything BUT with a calorie limit and/or macro guidelines so they don't become full binges.

The point of these days is to still get that calorie spike but without putting ourselves at risk for triggering a multi-day, or multi-week binge, like Cheat Days do for some people.

And Diet Breaks can help us bust through a plateau if we've been dieting for awhile. If you've been in a deficit for 3 or more months, and have already lost more than 10 pounds, you may want to consider a 1-2 week "break."

This break isn't an excuse to eat bad food. You still need to track. It is just a small calorie bump where you'll eat at more of a maintenance level. Usually about a 500 calorie bump works while still hitting your macros.

Regardless of which you ultimately decide to do, and you may find you use a combination of all three, go a few weeks when first starting out without ANYTHING.

Create a deficit and stay in it.

And if you want results as fast as possible, start with Macro Cheat Days only.

If you know cravings will destroy you if you don't get to indulge for too long, throw in some Cheat Days.

However, if you know a free-for-all day will mentally throw you off track, stick with Cheat Meals or Macro Cheat Days.

And especially if you have more weight to lose, wait to use a Diet Break until you've hit a plateau. A true plateau is when you haven't seen any results, despite changing your macro ratios, for 3-4 weeks.

If you are closer to your weight loss goals, and not a fan of Cheat Days or even Macro Cheat Days, you may consider adding in a Diet Break every 3-4 weeks, especially to up your training intensity for a couple of weeks!

Supplements For Weight Loss

There is no quick fix. No magic weight loss pill. So you can stop looking. Sorry to burst your bubble.

If you dial in your macros, you may find absolutely no supplements are even needed.

The only supplements I find to be super helpful for weight loss are protein powder and collagen because they can help you quickly and easily bump your protein intake.

Of course, whole, natural foods are always best, but sometimes having something we can reach for in a pinch helps.

And collagen can even be added to a morning cup of coffee or water during your workout!

If you are just starting back to your training routine, or even increasing your training intensity, you may also want to consider a BCAA supplement.

When we first start training, or increase our training frequency or intensity, we are much more likely to get sore from our sessions.

New moves and new workouts often cause us to be more sore. (Soreness is NOT an indicator that your workouts are good or hard enough...It is simply often due to doing something different.

But because we can get more sore and fatigued, adding in BCAAs may help. Studies have shown them to be helpful for reducing muscle soreness and speeding recovery in untrained individuals.

Another time to add in BCAAs may be if you choose to do Intermittent Fasting or train in a fasted state. Adding in BCAAs can promote protein synthesis and prevent muscle catabolism while in a fasted state. If you do use BCAAs during your fast, you need to consume UNFLAVORED BCAAs and add them to your water or coffee as flavored ones would break your fast.

Side note: Intermittent Fasting means you essential "skip" a meal. The most common form of IF is a 16 hour fast with an 8 hour eating window each day. And while meal timing is something you can adjust to fit your schedule, you should focus on truly eating when you're hungry. You don't have to force any specific meal timing.

Now what about fat burners?

The simple answer? I never recommend fat burners.

If you need an energy boost, drink coffee.

Change your meal timing and make sure you time more carbs right before and after your workout.

But fat burners are a waste of money. Not only do you adapt to the stimulant in them, so either need to keep consuming more to get the energy bump, or they don't really do anything.

Many are simply even caffeine, but with more crap added in so you'd be better off drinking coffee or tea.

And others have stimulants and ingredients that haven't been well tested.

For instance, Garcinia Cambogia, is a caffeine-free acidic fruit extract that has grown in popularity as a fat burner, but some studies have shown it may not be so good for your liver!

Just remember that if you do add in supplements, they need to remain supplemental!

Six Pack Macros: Focusing On Fat Loss

Dieting for abs...Some people will have an easier time with this than others. It just depends on where your natural set point is and where you tend to store body fat.

It also depends on how lean you are starting out.

I don't say this to discourage you from trying, but more to make it clear that getting a six pack or flat, defined, lean abs may take far more precision and dedication than simply losing weight.

It may take you reaching a level of leanness your body may initially want to fight against.

Simply even losing those last few pounds of fat is often a slower process than when we first started our weight loss journey.

So whether you want to lose those last few pounds of fat, or you really want to achieve washboard abs, these ratios and tips will help!

Where Do You Start?

The first thing to remember is - you can't out exercise a bad diet.

Often when we try to lose weight, we can see progress by simply changing up our workouts even if our diet isn't 100% dialed in.

Of course, long term we can't out exercise a bad diet, but simply increasing calorie expenditure to start can help.

But when it comes to reaching that new level of leanness and dropping those last few percentages of body fat so our abs show...

Don't even try it.

You can use your workouts to expedite your results, by including activation exercises prior to your interval workouts and compound lifts. This can allow you to use spot lipolysis to your advantage as much as possible (because every little bit doesn't hurt!), BUT there is no chance exercise alone is going to get you the fat loss results you want.

And for many of us to achieve abs, there is a need for not only dieting precision, but also consistency beyond what we are fully ready to commit to!

I Don't Want To Track...

Suck it up buttercup.

That's all I'm going to tell you.

Because when you want to achieve something that kind of goes against what your body really wants, you need to be precise.

Getting really lean is almost a science.

And to be precise you must track, weigh and measure everything. Vegetables aren't free foods.

Fiber counts.

It doesn't matter what dietary preference you follow, you'd better be ready to be exact in your portions.

Even those who've dieted for abs before, and understand the meals they need to eat, will still track.

I want to make this clear because I like to set people up for success and tracking is essential for results.

It's like if you want to make sure you wake up for that early morning flight, you freaking set an alarm....or maybe even two or three!

Even if it's close to the time you usually wake up, you set an alarm. You still want to GUARANTEE you'll make your flight.

That's the same reason you track and log and measure everything.

And be ready to do this CONSISTENTLY for longer than you'd like.

Because Guess What? Results Are Going To Be SLOW:

You can't rush fat loss.

It's not as simple as depleting your glycogen stores or losing water weight.

So if you want fast initial progress? It's just not going to happen.

If you drop your calories too low, you risk losing muscle and slowing your metabolic rate, which will cause your body to resist dropping more body fat.

Fat loss simply takes time.

And it may feel like nothing is happening when big results are actually occurring.

Working to get abs is going to test your patience.

Because you are at some point going to hit a "dead zone" where results are happening but you don't see any changes.

You may even feel like you look "worse" as stubborn areas seem to cling to the remaining fat while other areas lean down (and lean down only to the point of making you feel like the other areas look bigger!).

This phase is incredibly unsatisfying, BUT if you can hang in there, if you can TRUST THE PROCESS, all of the sudden it will feel like overnight you final notice a difference.

Embrace The Suck:

So I know I'm making achieving abs seem really attractive and fun (NOT!), but it can be amazing to push yourself to reach this goal if it's something you've always wanted!

It is almost like training for an athletic competition or sport...It's hard. It takes commitment on days we don't want to be committed.

And it takes us realizing we have to do things we don't always want to do!

We have to be prepared to get comfortable being uncomfortable.

Whether that means being the weirdo at parties not indulging in all of the treats, or whether that means cutting out foods we really LOVE because we know they will only serve to trigger further cravings, we have to learn to embrace the suck!

We need to commit to stricter ratios and realize that often when we want to eat unhealthy foods it is EMOTIONAL.

We don't really NEED those foods. We just WANT them.

They may add to our enjoyment at times and that is great, but we don't actually NEED them.

Now don't get me wrong, when we are maintaining and creating a lifestyle, we can totally indulge and find a balance. But if you want to achieve abs for the first time, it may mean saying BYE BYE to those treats for a bit!

So now that I've sold you on getting abs...

What Ratios Should You Use?

A calorie deficit alone isn't enough.

Macros matter most!

And I will tell you right now that for aesthetic goals, lower fat in general, is going to be key.

Fat has a minimal thermic effect, is very calorically dense and is not instant fuel for your workouts.

As long as you get enough for proper hormone functioning and health, you'll want to lower your fat intake first to create a calorie deficit.

Your carb intake will stay higher for longer as carbs help us prevent muscle catabolism by being the instant fuel our bodies need for our workouts. They spare our muscle tissue from being used as fuel instead.

Protein will also be kept high to help us retain lean muscle mass as we focus on losing fat.

So what macro ranges should you use?

Protein: High protein is key to promote protein synthesis and helps us make sure any weight we lose is fat. Protein should be kept between 40-50% of our daily calorie intake. This higher protein intake is key, especially if we are keeping up the intensity of our training, as muscle breakdown is elevated by being in a consistent calorie deficit.

Carbs: Your carb intake will range between 20-40% of your daily calories. You may go lower carb toward the end of your "cut" or as a first kickstart. While some people do respond better to lower carb, in general carbs should be kept higher as they are anti-catabolic. If you do lower them, make sure to time your carbs around your workouts!

Fat: Keeping fat intake between 20-35% is a great way to make sure you stay healthy while promoting fat loss as quickly as possible. For a kickstart or toward the end of your cut, you may drop your fat intake to between 10-15% of your calories, but do not keep it here for an extended period of time unless potentially boosting calories to a surplus.

What ratios can you use?

For fat loss and achieving that six pack, these are 5 great specific breakdowns to use and cycle:

-50% protein/30% carbs/20% fat
-40% protein/40% carbs/20% fat
-45% protein/30% carbs/25% fat
-45% protein/20% carbs/35% fat
-40% protein/30% carbs/30% fat

These ratios are all high protein and can be more challenging for people to hit.

This means you may have to spend more time planning to start. You may even want to do a two week kickstart before your true "cut" with a slightly lower protein ratio from the Weight Loss Macros section.

It is essential though that you hit these ratios within 2-3%. Precision is key for losing fat!

How should you cycle the ratios?

Planning ahead is key. You want to hit those ratios as closely as possible from that very first day.

And for fat loss, you'll want to cycle ratios every 1-2 weeks. These quicker changes can not only help mentally, because you can select different meals for each ratio, but they can also help you avoid hitting an extended plateau as there is often a "dead zone" when you're focused on losing fat.

Below are 2 different 6 week cycling options.

It is key you map out cycles for 4-6 weeks. This gives you an end date, which can be motivating and help you stay on track. It also gives you a date at which you can assess what you need to do next based on your progress.

Cycle #1 is for those looking to lose those last few pounds.

Cycle #2 is for those who want to get a six pack for the first time.

Cycle #1 - Lose Those Last Few Pounds:

To lose those last few pounds, stick with a ratio for 2 weeks at least for your first 6 week cycle. You may choose to go through this a second time if you aren't yet fully at your goal. If you do a second round, spend one week on each cycle and cycle through them twice.

For this cycle, you'll start with a more moderate carb and fat, but high protein ratio. The balance of carbs and fat to start should help you feel energized so you can keep training hard.

You'll then drop your carbs for only two weeks, as you increase your protein. This will accelerate your results without impacting your training for too long. You'll then increase carbs again to help fuel your training and protect your lean muscle mass.

Weeks 1-2: 40% protein/30% carbs/30% fat
Weeks 3-4: 45% protein/20% carbs/35% fat
Weeks 5-6: 45% protein/30% carbs/25% fat

Cycle #2 - Get That Six Pack!

These ratios may be more challenging to hit because of the very high protein levels. Mapping out sample days ahead of time and keeping meal prep simple will be key. Remember, this is a very specific goal and precision is key!

Fat will stay lower over the entire 6 week cycle. You will spend one week on a ratio before switching. After going through all 3 ratios, cycle back through, spending another week on each.

Starting with 45% protein and almost balanced carbs and fat should help you kickstart your results while staying fueled. It should also promote optimal hormone levels. You will cycle back through this slightly higher fat ratio on week 4 just to maintain hormonal balance even though the other levels are within that safe range.

On weeks 2 and 5, you'll drop your protein to the lowest points in this cycle and increase carbs for a little added energy boost. This should give your training a boost and help you not only protect your lean muscle, but potentially even gain muscle.

On weeks 3 and 6, you'll accelerate your results by bumping protein to 50%. This ratio will take more planning.

Also, make sure to up your water intake. Timing your carbs with protein around your workout will also be helpful, to keep your training intensity up.

Weeks 1 and 4: 45% protein/30% carbs/25% fat
Weeks 2 and 5: 40% protein/40% carbs/20% fat
Weeks 3 and 6: 50% protein/30% carbs/20% fat

Now...What About Daily Cycling Or Carb Cycling?

If you've been stalled for awhile and are close to your leanness goals, using a form of macro cycling, called carb cycling, may be the answer!

It can help you keep your training intensity higher while taking advantage of both higher carb and lower carb ratios!

The daily cycling can help you kickstart your progress when you've stalled, especially when going lower calorie is not an option. Be prepared to really plan things out ahead of time and do some extra meal prep work though!

If you choose to cycle daily you'll want to use this simple set up. Set your protein at one gram per pound of bodyweight each day and then set carbs at 20% of your calories on low carb days and 50% of your calories on high carb days.

The leftover calories will be fat.

You will also want to potentially cycle your calories if you do this. Cycling your calories can help you kickstart your results, without creating more of a deficit.

For example, if you want to average about 1500 calories per day based on your calculations, you will then want to set calories at about 1300 on low carb, or non training days, and 1700 on high carb or training days.

You will then want to calculate 1 gram per pound of current bodyweight and subtract those calories first. Then calculate your carbs after (20% on low carb days or 50% on high carb days) and whatever is leftover will be your fat intake.

While I do mention lowering carbs and calories on non-training days while raising calories and carbs on training days, you may find you do need to adjust the schedule based on when you train each day.

You may also find that TIMING your carbs on low carb days to later at night, if you train in the morning, is super helpful.

If you train intensely multiple days in a row, instead of alternating higher and lower days, you could do 3-4 days lower carb and then one day higher carb.

And this way you can put your hardest training sessions, or the workouts for those muscles you'd like to grow, on those higher carb days or right after them.

While carb cycling is complicated and not necessary for most of us, it can be something to consider when you've hit a plateau in your fat loss efforts for 3-4 weeks. Just note, energy levels can fluctuate dramatically because of the constant changes in carbs.

How Many Calories Should You Eat?

To push your body past its set point, and for those cutting for a competition, you may hit some more extreme calorie deficits.

But this is NOT where you want to start.

Often creating LESS of a deficit and staying consistent for longer will lead to far better results.

Fat loss is slower than weight loss because your focus is on ONLY losing fat. Often with weight loss we are more accepting of some muscle mass being lost, especially when we have more weight to lose to start.

But you need to be more cautious with creating a bigger calorie deficit the leaner you are because the body's response to calorie deprivation makes it easy to rebound and regain all of the weight you've lost.

When we create large calorie deficits, our metabolism adapts and "slows" down. Plus often, we lose as much muscle as we do fat only further stalling our results. And if that wasn't bad enough, the extreme deficit can make your body think it's starving.

When you then fall off of your diet, which is easy to do when your body is telling you that you're "starving," you'll not only regain the weight you once lost, but often end up with worse body composition than where you started. You unfortunately don't regain the muscle mass you lost when your weight rebounds.

So while you want to create a calorie deficit, do not go below 11 x goal bodyweight (which may be your current weight) especially to start.

If you've been relatively lean for awhile, but need that final push to get your abs to show, you may want to consider even 13-14 x goal bodyweight. This may put you in enough of a deficit without your training suffering.

You do also need to make sure your deficit fits your ratio. With some of the higher protein ratios, like the one at 50%, you may find you need more calories to actually get better results!

Another thing to consider when planning out your calorie intake is whether you will include a Diet Break or Macro Cheat Day. Note, I did not mention Cheat Days as you will want to abstain from full free-for-alls when first trying to get a six pack.

The more you plan in calorie spikes, like a Diet Break or Macro Cheat, the more you will want to create a deficit on other days to balance everything out.

Should You Include Cheat Days, Macro Cheat Days Or Diet Breaks?

When trying to get abs, Cheat Days are basically a no-go. Maybe you have one every 4 to 6 weeks, but overall, you need consistency day in and day out.

Macro Cheat Days, with strategic boosts in carbs and calories, may be used to help you stay fueled for your workouts.

For these strategic spikes, you will want to limit the spike to about 500 calories and focus simply on boosting carbs. While this may cause you to gain weight on the scale, it is temporary. You will want to do these only 2-4 times a month at most.

They can also be a great mental break if you feel yourself needing one!

And Diet Breaks, may be key if you've hit a plateau or even mentally need the break from being in a constant deficit. It is better to strategically bump your calories for a couple of weeks by 500 than to binge or fall off your plan.

The consistency needed to get abs and the constant deficit isn't easy.

To have hit a plateau worthy of a Diet Break, you have to have stalled for 3-4 weeks. If you're a woman, a plateau of less than that length could be because of hormone fluctuations.

But if you've not seen changes for 3-4 weeks while being precise and consistent with your nutrition (and you have logs to verify), a Diet Break may be just what you need to push yourself over the hump.

Supplements For Fat Loss

Supplements can be helpful at this stage of dieting as everything else should already be dialed in.

BCAAs and creatine can help you build and retain muscle while in a deficit.

While we don't want to rely on supplements, at the end of a cut, caffeine, creatine and BCAAs (NOT pre-workout stimulants) can all help you power through an intense training session and speed your recovery.

All of these things can help you get better results from your training while being in an extended calorie deficit.

It is essential we work on retaining our lean muscle mass if we want that sexy, strong lean look to go with our six pack abs!

Plus, more muscle means a "healthier" metabolism and more calories burned even at rest aka better and faster fat loss results!

Protein powders and collagen are two other key supplements that can really help you hit those super high protein ratios that lead to faster results.

Does Meal Timing Matter?

If you hit your calories and macros overall for the day, you're going to get results no matter what your goals are.

But when fat loss is your goal, manipulating your meal timing CAN help make things easier.

While doing intermittent fasting, can work just as well as 6 small meals a day, the key is making sure you're timing your food to help you get the most out of your workouts.

Because of the calorie deficit, if you aren't training fasted in the morning, it will be key to get carbs and protein right before and after your workouts. Save your fats for meals not close to your training.

Even getting EXTRA protein and a good chunk of your carbs right post workout can help aid in your recovery and create a more anabolic environment.

If you are training fasted in the morning, BCAAs can come in handy during your workouts and you will want to consume more carbs before bed. You do not need to fear eating carbs before bed, especially if you train early in the morning and are in a consistent deficit!

While meal timing can be adjusted to fit your schedule, at this stage, paying a bit more attention to fueling pre and post workout can help!

One Last Thing…Is It Worth It?

You don't need a six pack to feel and look good. You can feel and look amazing at any weight!

Abs don't make you better or more worthwhile or more beautiful.

A six pack can be something you desire, but your worth can't be wrapped up in getting it.

Dieting for abs is like training for a race or competition - it is a specific goal and a challenge to conquer.

But you can't constantly be training for race after race or you'll burn out. You have to have "off seasons."

And dieting for abs is the same way.

You aren't really creating a lifestyle, but instead are working toward that one specific goal.

And that is a-ok.

But you will need an "exit" strategy for after you get lean. You need an "off season" routine.

This can mean shifting your focus to building muscle or even to simply maintaining your hard work.

We will always be a work in progress, just make sure you appreciate the journey!

Muscle Macros

Not every "diet" is about eating less or losing weight.

Sometimes we want to GAIN, especially gain MUSCLE!

Strong is the new sexy, haven't you heard!?

What if you want to lose fat though as you gain muscle?

While many of us have heard this isn't possible...it actually IS possible!

It's just a slower process. And to get the best results possible, you do want to make one or the other your main focus.

Especially if you are just starting your weight loss journey, and have more than 5-10 pounds to lose, make weight loss your primary goal.

If you are within your ideal weight range though, you can shift your focus to adding muscle even if you would still like to get leaner.

It's important to note that the process of building muscle does require you to eat in a surplus. And this can result in weight being gained on the scale.

This doesn't mean you're going to "get fat."

But often people struggle to gain muscle because they don't allow themselves to actually eat enough for growth.

They fear seeing that number on the scale go up.

So if you're serious about gaining muscle, either ditch the scale or just be prepared to see that number increase!

However, there are ways to minimize fat gain as you add muscle, especially if you commit to a slower, and "cleaner," bulk.

Start By Creating A Calorie Surplus

Your body needs fuel to grow. This means eating more than you burn.

Start with a calorie calculation of 14-15x goal bodyweight (which may be your current bodyweight) and listen to your body to increase from there.

You want to really make sure your workouts feel good and that you're refueling with a big snack after.

Also, set a calorie range for yourself of even 200-300 calories plus or minus.

While unused energy will be stored as fat, often a surplus of at least 1,000 calories over our maintenance intake is required to create muscle growth, especially if you've been training for awhile and aren't just starting back.

Just remember that, while you want a surplus, this isn't an excuse to eat everything in sight. If you overeat too much, you will gain fat.

A bigger surplus doesn't mean more muscle growth.

And gaining too much fat can be detrimental to your progress too. As you gain fat, insulin sensitivity drops and so do testosterone levels.

If you become more insulin resistant, protein synthesize can be suppressed and your ability to burn fat decreases. This means it becomes harder to gain muscle and easier to gain fat.

Also, when your testosterone levels drop, your estrogen levels increase. This can promote fat storage and make it harder to build muscle.

This is why with your calorie surplus you really want to mind your macros!

Using Those Macro Ratios To Gain Muscle

By not just eating everything in sight, and by hitting specific macro breakdowns, you can stay leaner as you gain muscle.

You can also help yourself crush your workouts and see major increases on your lifts!

There can be some amazing performance benefits from using the high carb ratios that will also help you gain muscle.

Carbs are key for gaining muscle as they promote a more anabolic environment in your body and can help improve your recovery.

When you restrict carbs, your muscle glycogen levels drop and low glycogen stores can inhibit signaling related to post-workout muscle repair and growth.

While you can get away with not working out when you want to lose weight, you can't gain muscle if you don't train. To gain muscle, you need to do some sort of resistance training, even if those workouts use only your own bodyweight.

When training hard, restricting your carbs can raise cortisol levels and lower testosterone levels which will affect your recovery.

Low carb diets can also decrease strength and muscular endurance, making it harder to create progressive overload in your workouts, and hindering maximal muscle growth.

So for this reason, I recommend higher carb ratios.

So what macro ranges should you use?

Protein: Protein should still be kept higher to promote optimal muscle growth while also preventing you from gaining fat. Keep your protein intake between 30-45% of your calories. Generally staying in that 30-40% range is more than enough; however, if you've been dieting down or cutting fat, you may want to start with your protein slightly higher as you first increase your calorie intake.

Carbs: Carbs are key to fuel your workouts and aid in muscle growth. Keep carbs between 35-50% of your daily calorie intake. You want your glycogen stores full so reducing cardio can be helpful too. But if you do still plan to run or keep in more cardio activities, you may find you need to keep your carbs between 40-50%.

Fat: Fat intake will be kept lower although you don't want to drop below 20% and risk hormonal imbalances. Keeping your fat intake between 20-30% will help you maintain your health while focusing your diet on carbs and protein!

What ratios should you use?

A lower fat diet works well when you're looking to gain muscle.
While you want to make sure you have enough fat to create ideal hormone levels, you do want your focus to be on carbs.

And by also keeping your protein intake higher, you can prevent extra fat gain.

For gaining muscle, these are 5 great specific breakdowns to use and cycle:

-40% protein/40% carbs/20% fat
-30% protein/40% carbs/30% fat
-35% protein/45% carbs/20% fat
-30% protein/50% carbs/20% fat
-45% protein/35% carbs/20% fat

How should you cycle the ratios?

Longer cycles, so a longer time spent on each ratio, works well when you're trying to gain. Spending 3-6 weeks on each ratio allows you to change ratios with your workout progression.

Changing ratios can help you avoid gaining extra fat and even allow you to adjust based on changes to your workout routine so you're always fueled.

Below are 2 different 9 week cycling options. I recommend adjusting these so you change ratios with a change in your workout progression.

Cycle #1 is for those purely focused on gaining muscle.

Cycle #2 is for those who would rather gain slower to really avoid gaining fat.

Cycle #1 - Pure Muscle Gains:

If you're training intense, and even want to keep more cardio in your routine, these ratios will fuel that activity while promoting muscle growth.

They are also perfect for anyone that struggles to add muscle or who's been lean for awhile so only wants to focus on building.

Your protein will remain just high enough to promote a cleaner bulk while the higher carb intake will really fuel muscle growth by creating that anabolic environment ideal for protein synthesis.

By cycling your fat intake up for a 3 week period in the middle, you'll also help maintain optimal hormone levels and health.

Cycle ratios every 3 weeks, or with your workout progression. Do not exceed 6 weeks on a ratio. And you may even switch them more frequently if you find your results have slowed and you're starting to gain more fat.

Weeks 1-3: 30% protein/50% carbs/20% fat
Weeks 4-6: 30% protein/40% carbs/30% fat
Weeks 7-9: 35% protein/45% carbs/20% fat

Cycle #2 - Gain Muscle Without The Fat:

If you've struggled to fully commit in the past to gaining muscle because you're worried about gaining a ton of fat, this 9 week cycle is a great place to start.

These higher protein ratios can help you stay leaner and even build without as much of a calorie surplus. These lower fat ratios will also help prevent excess fat gain while your higher carb intake will promote muscle growth.

Especially if you're coming off of a cut, starting with the highest protein intake first can help you transition to the calorie surplus without gaining fat. You'll then lower protein and increase carbs to expedite your gains before cycling your protein back up to help you potentially lose any extra fat you've gained while still adding muscle!

Cycle these ratios every 3 weeks for a 9 week cycle. While you can extend out each cycle, 3 weeks is best to avoid gaining fat.

Weeks 1-3: 45% protein/35% carbs/20% fat
Weeks 4-6: 35% protein/45% carbs/20% fat
Weeks 7-9: 40% protein/40% carbs/20% fat

Should You Include Cheat Days, Macro Cheat Days Or Diet Breaks?

Part of the benefit of Cheat Days, Macro Cheat Days and Diet Breaks is the calorie spike. It's also a day to indulge in foods that may not be as easy to fit in while we are calorie restricted and hitting our macros.

So while you don't need any of these for a calorie spike during a muscle gaining cycle, you may designate certain days as Cheat Days or Macro Cheat Days for "mental" purposes.

Because the quality of your food does matter, and eating more whole, natural foods will get you better results, you may decide to avoid certain foods on your average day.

So having one day designated as the day you indulge in those more processed treats can be a great way to find balance.

However, if you do include a Cheat Day, try to keep within your normal surplus while not caring about your macro breakdown.

You can also do a Macro Cheat Day, hitting your ratio and calories while simply not caring about food quality.

Cheat Meals are potentially the best option when you're in a calorie surplus because you can have one "lower quality" meal that you've "saved up" calories for while still remaining within your calorie range and even your macros for the day.

With just a meal, you can make sure to still fuel properly around your workouts to fully benefit from your training sessions.

You just want to be careful with these days as you are already in a calorie surplus!

You will not need a Diet Break when you're in a surplus. Although, you can always do a quick 1-2 week "cut" if you do find you're gaining some fat. This is the reverse of a Diet Break, and you'd actually just lower calories for a 1-2 week period.

Supplements For Gaining Muscle

With a calorie surplus, it is easy to get everything you need from whole, natural foods.

So while you never "need" supplements, creatine and protein powder can be two go-tos when gaining muscle, especially if they make things easier.

BCAAs during your workout may also be added, especially if you're training fasted, but can be a waste of money otherwise since you're eating enough protein and carbs to promote muscle growth and recovery.

What is creatine?

Creatine is a mixture of 3 important amino acids glycine, arginine, and methionine and does exist naturally within our bodies.

The supplement is often a flavorless powder that you mix with water during your workout.

You can get creatine through foods such as red meat and fish, which means you can get enough through whole, natural foods, especially if you eat meat.

If you don't eat meat, are older or even female, you may find a creatine supplement helpful!

Creatine is meant to help fuel our muscles and produce energy quickly, which means it can boost our performance in the gym.

Creatine is best taken with a carb source to raise insulin levels and optimize creatine uptake into your muscles. It can be taken pre or post workout, but is most often recommended to be used within one hour of exercise.

One "risk" of creatine is weight gain.

Part of the reason for potential weight gain with creatine is water retention. It is key you drink enough water to ensure proper cellular hydration.

How Does Creatine Help With Muscle Gains?

Creatine boosts our performance in the gym. And we can't gain muscle if we aren't able to train hard.

Creatine helps:

-Increase strength and power
-Increase work capacity
-Reduce fatigue

Creatine can improve our strength and power because it serves as an energy reserve for the body during short, intense bouts of exercise. It literally increases energy levels in your muscles by increasing phosphocreatine, which leads to an increase in ATP production. And ATP is the energy supply you need to work harder and improve your strength and power output.

It can also increase your work capacity, which means you can do a larger volume of work without fatiguing.

And because of the improvements in your power, strength and work capacity with creatine, you can trainer harder and get more out of your training sessions.

This can lead to better muscle gains without you gaining fat!

Another interesting thing to note with creatine supplementation is the difference that men and women can see in their results.

Men tend to see bigger muscle gains while women may actually see more body fat lost from adding in a creatine supplement.

While creatine may be the right fit for you, and can have amazing benefits especially if you don't eat meat, you can get sufficient amounts from red meat and fish!

It may also be more beneficial for us as we get older and struggle to retain lean muscle mass.

Just remember we always want to focus on whole, natural foods first.

So if you choose to add in this supplement, make sure to track how it affects you!

The Proper Pairing:

While you can't out exercise a bad diet to lose weight, you can't gain muscle without a proper training routine.

Focusing on strength training, and yes bodyweight workouts can count, is key if you want to build muscle.

And if you're doing a ton of cardio, you're going to fight against your muscle gaining efforts. Especially if you're doing a ton of steady-state cardio.

Those endurance activities are more catabolic to muscle tissue and will often deplete your glycogen stores more quickly! They can also fatigue you for your lifting sessions.

So if you do include cardio, lowering the intensity of your sessions or keeping it to shorter bouts after your strength workouts can be helpful.

And while you want to use a variety of rep and set ranges, including some maximal strength work can help you get better results faster.

If you want to gain muscle, you need to focus your workouts on strength and hypertrophy for the most part!

Recovery in between sessions is key too.

You don't want to over exercise in an attempt to try to get results faster.

Sufficient rest during your workouts between lifts, and also between training sessions, may matter almost as much as the weights you actually lift!

Less rest or more training sessions isn't always better.

So start tracking your workouts as well as your nutrition if you want to get killer muscle gains!

Maintenance Macros

You've lost the weight you wanted to lose. You've gained the muscle you wanted to gain.

Now what?!

How do you maintain the results you've worked so hard to get?

Because all too often we reach our goal only to fall back into old habits. Old habits that land us right back where we started.

Maintaining the progress we've made, to start at least, can be a challenge.

Because we can't just return to what we were doing BEFORE we started the diet.

So how can you maintain the progress you've made?

How can you find a balance where you can maintain your results, but also gain a bit more freedom?

Where Do You Start?

There are two main ways to start transitioning into more of a maintenance phase.

The first way is to start by slowly adjusting calories as you continue on with the ratio you've been using.

This way you're making one change at a time and monitoring your intake to avoid gaining fat or losing muscle.

The second way is to keep your calories about the same while adjusting to more of a moderate macro ratio.

If you've been on a ratio that is much higher in one of the macros, you may transition to something more along the lines of 35% protein/33% carbs/32% fat (basically 35% protein and your carbs and fat about even).

This way you are still helping yourself avoid unnecessary fat gain while protecting your hard earned muscle mass, but you are also creating a more balanced approach that can allow you more freedom with your food choices.

The key is to not just revert back to old habits but to have an "exit" strategy.

It means finding a maintainable balance that keeps you full and fueled but also helps you retain your results.

And while there WILL be fluctuations, times you gain or lose because you're more or less dedicated, you want a baseline to return to so that you don't end back in the yo-yo dieting cycle!

How Many Calories Should You Eat?

Most of the time when we talk about our calorie intake, we are either discussing how to create a deficit or a surplus.

Let's face it, we most often consider dietary changes when we want to lose or gain weight. We rarely consider what we then need to do to maintain those results.

This is where a range will come in handy as you learn what your body now needs since achieving your goals.

Transitioning From A Weight Loss Or Fat Loss Cycle:

If you've lost weight, your energy expenditure may have gone down.

It often increases over time as you maintain your results, but it is important to note that initially, you may feel like you need to keep your calories slightly lower.

By focusing on macros during weight loss, you can avoid severe metabolic adaptation and muscle mass loss.

But you will still slowly need to "retrain" your body to eat more.

Increasing your training intensity coming out of the deficit can be helpful. And with increasing your calories, it may be easy and even fun to do!

Being more active in general as you transition into a maintenance phase can be helpful. So find fun activities to do so that you can keep your metabolism running strong.

And consider slowly bumping your daily calorie intake by 100-200.

Increase every couple of weeks until you hit a point where you consistently feel satisfied from your meals. Note I didn't say "full" because full denotes overeating. Your energy should be consistent, your workouts should feel fueled, and you shouldn't be really gaining or losing, but staying in a consistent range with your weight.

You want to slowly increase calories so you can monitor what your body needs. To give yourself a range to shoot for after weight loss, maintenance is usually between 12-13x current bodyweight to start.

If you were more active throughout your weight loss or fat loss phase, and if you've really increased your training intensity as you've come out of the deficit, you may even find you increase to 13-14x current bodyweight.

Transitioning From A Muscle Building Cycle:

If you've added muscle, your caloric needs will have increased. However, you don't need to maintain the surplus you've been in to build.

Slowly lowering your daily calorie intake by 100-200 calories is a good place to start. Make changes slowly every week or so.

You may even find you cycle your calories based on your training that day, going slightly higher on harder training days and slightly lower on easier workouts or off days.

You may even keep a higher calorie day solely on one training day. If you do this, keep the "surplus" on the day of your hardest workout or on the day you train your most "stubborn" muscle group. You'll then drop calories lower on the other days.

You just want your calories to average out over the week to a 100-200 drop below your surplus.

Often if you've built muscle, you'll find a calorie intake between 13-15x current bodyweight works well.

For some of us, our "surplus" may no longer be that much of a surplus, especially as we change up our ratios, even lowering our carb intake.

Just make sure to adjust your calories slowly so that your training doesn't suffer, focusing still on timing more calories right around your workouts!

What Macro Ratios Should You Use To Maintain?

When you first transition into a maintenance phase, you may want to stick with the ratios in your previous cycle as you first adjust calories.

This can help us mentally feel better about the changes - it can feel "safer" and less like we are risking losing everything we worked hard for, especially after a weight loss phase.

One of the hardest parts about adjusting our diet is the feeling that we may "lose it all" and end up right back where we started.

This is why small, slow adjustments, where you continue to track, are key.

Once you've been maintaining for even just 6-8 weeks, you may find you feel comfortable enough to log and track more loosely.

But to start, to help guarantee results, you need to track and monitor your transition.

So while you can stay with the ratio cycle you were doing as you adjust calories first, you can also maintain closer to your current calorie intake as you adjust to a more moderate macro ratio.

Even simply adjusting macros can help you start to transition into retaining the results you've worked hard for.

So what macro ranges should you use?

While you may find you really enjoyed a specific ratio you already did, and go back to that, generally we'll want to do a ratio that more evenly divides our calories in thirds.

Protein: Generally, you will still want to keep protein high as you transition. Between 30-40% can help you avoid muscle mass loss or unnecessary fat gain. The longer you've spent "maintaining" your results, the more you may find you only need about 25% protein to stay at your new set point.

Carbs: Here is where you have some flexibility based on your training and any changes you are making to your routine. You can go lower carb if you find you enjoy fats more and feel better on higher fat. Or you can go higher carb if you feel better doing that and are increasing your training intensity further. Coming off a weight loss or fat loss phase, you may want to keep carbs close to what you were doing because increasing carbs could cause weight gain on the scale due to changes in your glycogen stores and water retention. A range between 20-40% works well, unless you're starting to train for an endurance sport.

Fat: Just like with carbs, there is some flexibility to how much fat you consume. If you've been in a lower fat cycle, going through at least a 2-3 week phase of slightly higher fat can be helpful to promote an optimal balance in your body. Especially if you've cut fats to the lowest level during a fat loss phase, a period of higher fat can be key. Your fat intake will be in the 25-45% range.

What ratios should you use?

Unless you really enjoy low carb or low fat specifically, or unless you're training for an endurance sport, generally the more balanced all 3 macros are, the easier it is to stick to a plan consistently while maintaining your results.

Ratios that are more moderate are a great way to focus on creating a balance.

Again, the longer you've maintained your results, the more flexibility you will find you have in the exact macros you use. And you may even find you track more loosely because you can more intuitively eat the portions you need.

But to start, making sure protein is still the star can be key!

More moderate ratios to start your Maintenance Phase are:

-35% protein/33% carbs/32% fat
-40% protein/30% carbs/30% fat
-30% protein/40% carbs/30% fat
-30% protein/30% carbs/40% fat
-30% protein/35% carbs/35% fat

The key is selecting ratios that allow for incremental changes from your current cycle, even if you decide to stick with those other ratios at first as you adjust calories.

How should you cycle ratios?

When you're maintaining your current results, you have much more flexibility in the length of your cycles. You may choose to only switch them when you switch up your workout progressions.

Even though you aren't working toward anything specifically, still cycling every 5-6 weeks can help you avoid losing any of the progress you've worked hard to build.

These changes in ratios can even allow for mini muscle building or fat loss phases so that you never really have to do extended cuts or bulks.

Below are two cycles you can use as you first transition to help you strike a balance.

Cycle #1 is a great transition from a weight loss or fat loss phase.

Cycle #2 is a perfect way to transition from a muscle building phase.

Cycle #1 - Transitioning From A Fat Loss Or Weight Loss Phase:

Start with 1-2 weeks on the first ratio so you're more closely monitoring how things are going and can switch ratios as needed to help avoid any "backsliding." You can then slowly increase the length of time you spend on each ratio.

And when you find something you really enjoy, even consider 6 straight weeks there.

Over these weeks, protein will decrease as fats increase.

Week 1-2: 40% protein/30% carbs/30% fat
Week 3-5: 35% protein/33% carbs/32% fat
Week 6-9: 30% protein/30% carbs/40% fat

Cycle #2 - Transitioning From A Muscle Building Phase:

Just like with transitioning from a fat loss or weight loss phase, start with 1-2 weeks on the first ratio you select so you're more closely monitoring how things are going and can switch ratios as needed to help avoid any "backsliding." You can then slowly increase the length of time you spend on each ratio.

And when you find something you really enjoy, even consider 6 straight weeks there.

Over these weeks, your carb intake will decrease and settle in a moderate range, especially compared to many of the ratios you were on during a surplus.

Week 1-2: 30% protein/40% carbs/30% fat
Week 3-5: 30% protein/35% carbs/35% fat
Week 6-9: 35% protein/33% carbs/32% fat (you may even choose to lower carbs here to 30%)

Should You Include Cheat Days, Macro Cheat Days Or Diet Breaks?

You shouldn't need a set Diet Break during this period as that is essential what maintenance is - a break from any specific dieting goal.

But since you aren't working toward anything specific, both Cheat Days and Macro Cheat Days can be used as you see fit to strike a lifestyle balance.

Just know that the bigger these spikes are, and the more frequent they are, the more that will affect your overall weekly calorie intake.

So if you do too many huge spikes while eating higher calorie during the week already, you can end up gaining weight.

The more calorie spikes you include, the lower your maintenance calories during the week may be to find a balance so you don't end up in that yo-yo dieting cycle.

However, this doesn't mean you should starve yourself during the week to be able to do a massive Cheat Day.

This can cause negative metabolic adaptations, which can cause you to struggle to maintain your results.

So starting out, as you increase your calories and adjust your ratios, you may find a Cheat Meal or Macro Cheat Day is better for you.

But this is why it is also key to continue to track as you transition!

Supplements For Maintenance

I recommend continuing to use any supplements you've been taking as you first transition. Over time you may find you remove all supplements or simply keep in ones that make hitting your macros easier.

Many people will continue to use protein supplements and collagen.

If you are also coming out of a weight loss or fat loss phase, you may start to use, or continue to use, BCAAs as well. These can help if you're increasing your training intensity as they can improve your recovery.

Creatine will also be something you'll most likely stop using after your muscle building phase. Unless you are a Vegetarian, or struggling to retain lean muscle mass, due to age, you won't necessarily want to continue using it.

Plus, some cycling of creatine can be helpful.

Now What About Tracking? Do I Have To Do It Forever?!

Tracking isn't fun. While it becomes easier, and you may not even really think about it now, it's never really something you want to do.

Any time you want results, you NEED to track to help yourself guarantee you're doing the right things to get those results. But as you adjust to a "lifestyle," tracking isn't as necessary.

Tracking as you first transition can help you avoid the all too common yo-yo dieting cycle that occurs.

We lose the weight or make the change only to slip back into old habits that completely erase all of our hard work.

So tracking to start can help us avoid that.

But as you start to find a routine, you may find you don't need to track to hit your ratios.

Before you just completely stop logging though, you may find it helpful to just monitor your protein intake. Only log the protein that you eat to make sure you're eating enough. Just this little acknowledgment of what you're consuming can be helpful.

From there, you may set periods where you do a "check in," logging for a few days or even a week just to monitor your consumption. You may especially do this at points where you adjust ratios even with your workout routine.

But over time, no, you do not need to track as strictly!

Endurance Sport Macros

CARBS!

When we think about training for an endurance sport, we think about carb loading.

As an endurance runner or cyclist, you may even think you'll die of exhaustion on the spot if you don't get enough carbs.

But often we overestimate our carb needs, which can not only be detrimental to our training, but can even lead to weight gain despite all of the hours spent working out.

You may find that very first race you train for, the weight seems to fall off. It's because you've increased your energy expenditure.

But you may notice that over your training you hit a plateau. Or that as you build up for that next race, you don't seem to be getting the same weight loss benefits.

And that's often because our bodies have adapted to the steady-state cardio training.

This can cause us to be faced with the difficult question of....

Do I focus on fueling my runs or rides for my race? Or do I focus on losing weight?

But it doesn't have to be either or! You just need to plan based on your training routine and your level of training "experience."

Beginners May Need MORE Than Experienced Racers

The reason you get stronger and can run or ride further faster is because your body adapts. It becomes more efficient.

However, because your body adapts to your long runs or rides, you actually need fewer calories to fuel you.

Your calorie requirements, and even your carb requirements, may go down, but this doesn't mean you should eat less and less.

Actually eating less may lead to more muscle catabolism, worse training sessions and even metabolic adaptation.

It's just important that we understand we may need to fuel differently based on our training experience.

Experienced runners or cyclists may actually be way more efficient so their caloric and carb needs may be lower.

The long distance runs aren't as much of a "shock" to their bodies as when they were a newbie racer!

That is why to start, you may see quick weight loss results with these cardio workouts but also a quicker, and sometimes even sudden, plateau.

Just remember it's because you've adapted, and adaptation is what allows us to run further faster!

Beginners, do not be afraid to bump your calories a bit higher when you're first starting out, even if you also want to lose weight. This can even help you prevent muscle catabolism from the steady-state cardio!

Cycling Your Diet With Your Training

You plan out your training routine so you don't peak before your race. And you'll want to do the exact same thing with your diet.

While weight loss can be a "benefit" of training for a race, you need to focus on one main goal.

If weight loss is your main goal, you may want to select one of the higher carb weight loss ratios with a slightly more active calorie calculation, especially if it is your first race.

But if you want to set a PR or train to complete that longer race you've never done before, you need your diet to be focused on fueling your performance FIRST.

You can then adjust your macros based on the length of your race, where you are in your training program and even if you are in season or out of season.

What Ratios Should You Use?

Too often our ratios are far too carb heavy way before we actually need those extra carbs as fuel.

Remember, if you don't use the energy, you store it as fat.

Also, running longer distances, or doing steady-state cardio in general, can be catabolic to muscle tissue.

Because it is harder to retain lean muscle mass with endurance sports, not only do you often need to increase your calories, but you also need more protein.

Going higher protein will help promote protein synthesis so you can retain your lean muscle mass and run or ride faster further. This can also help you get, and stay, lean.

And if you did any off season lifting, it will make sure you retain those gains as your runs or rides increase in length!

So what macro ranges should you use?

Protein: Often endurance athletes get so focused on more carbs that they don't consume enough protein. And this is part of the reason why endurance sports are often catabolic to muscle tissue. Keeping your protein between 30-40% for most of your training program will be key, especially if you are a more experienced racer. You may find that the last few weeks right before your race, you increase carbs further, dropping protein to 25% of your intake.

Carbs: While carbs an important fuel source, you don't get added benefits from eating more than you need. Actually this can hinder your progress because you'll most likely gain weight. Only as you increase miles should your carb intake really increase. For most of your training you may find between 30-40% of your calories coming from carbs is more than enough. As you get toward that final 4-6 weeks of training, you may then increase to 50% or even 55% of your calories coming from carbs.

Fat: You want enough fat to promote optimal hormone functioning. This is especially important for female endurance athletes as missed periods, and even no periods, are more common among the endurance athlete community. To keep optimal hormone levels, keep your fat around 30% for a good part of your training, dropping no lower than 20% as you get closer and closer to your race.

What ratios should you use?

With training for a race, you will want to cycle ratios based on increases in mileage. You want to make sure you're fueling your training as it becomes more intense.

Below are 4 ratios that work well for endurance athletes. You may find you cycle between all 4 as you get closer to your race or you may find you only use 2 or 3 of them.

In your off season, you may even want to consider using the ratios in the Muscle Macros section to help you add lean muscle to power your runs or rides.

Gaining muscle isn't just for body builders! It can simply be about becoming stronger for your runs or rides!

Use these 4 ratios over the course of your training plan to be in peak shape for your race:

-40% protein/30% carbs/30% fat
-30% protein/40% carbs/30% fat
-30% protein/50% carbs/20% fat
-25% protein/55% carbs/20% fat

You'll notice that all are higher carb ratios and increase in carbs as you get closer to your race week.

Unless you know your body does really well on low carb, I would not recommend high fat ratios if you are a serious runner or cyclist. If you do decide to experiment with lower carb, don't do it during your peak training season.

How should you cycle ratios?

Stick with one ratio for 2-4 weeks. You want to change ratios as your training intensifies but you also want a consistent source of energy.

You may find that as you get closer to your race, you only spend 1 week on that final ratio. Having a "peak week" routine is never bad especially as you focus on winding down to be ready.

Using the ratios in this order is generally best. However, if your race is shorter, you may find that you stick with just the first two ratios and don't need to go above that 40% carb intake.

Week 1-4: 40% protein/30% carbs/30% fat
Week 5-7: 30% protein/40% carbs/30% fat
Week 8-10: 30% protein/50% carbs/20% fat
Week 11-12: 25% protein/55% carbs/20% fat

Remember you do not need to use all of the ratios for every training routine but setting up a diet plan to match your training will get you even better results!

How Many Calories Do You Need?

You will want to cycle calories, increasing your intake as the intensity of your training goes up.

I also highly recommend giving yourself a daily range so that, while you may not intentionally cycle, you don't feel "guilty" indulging in more calories on days your runs or rides did take a toll. This can also allow you to cycle down if you aren't as hungry on a non-training day or even as you start to adapt more to the intensity of your routine.

Again, your body ADAPTS. It's why runs get easier, which is a good thing, BUT it also means we need to consume fewer calories because we are more efficient and burning less.

Set a range between 200 calories plus or minus. Do not conscious ADD in the calories from your workouts, but don't be afraid to respond to hunger from them.

To start, set your calories between 12-15 x goal bodyweight (which may be your CURRENT weight).

This is a wide range because it will also be dependent on your experience level and ultimate goal.

Beginners who haven't been training and are just starting out, may be able to do 13-14x goal bodyweight. If their goal is weight loss, they may even be able to do 12 x goal bodyweight, but I do not recommend going lower.

Experienced exercisers that are already lean, may find that 13-15 x current bodyweight works well depending on the length of the race they are training for.

If you want to focus more on weight loss, but have been competing in an endurance sport for awhile, you may find you actually need to keep your protein higher and set your calorie intake at about 12-13 x goal bodyweight to lose fat as you train.

Just remember that under fueling can be as detrimental as over fueling.

Instead of just turning to more carbs when you need energy, think about increasing your overall calorie intake.

If you don't eat enough calories, you can feel low energy and sluggish during your runs or rides and even cause more muscle catabolism.

Tracking Is Key

With your runs or rides you track how they felt, what distances you did, and even the time it took you to complete them so you can improve on your results.

And if you want to get the most out of your training, you also need to understand how your diet impacts your performance.

That is why it is so important to track and log your nutrition, whether you're an experienced runner or cyclist looking to constantly improve or simply looking to lose weight as you train.

If you PR in a race, don't you want to be able to replicate and improve on those results?

Then you need a log of everything you did, including how you fueled.

If you constantly want to improve, you need to track everything so you know exactly what works and what doesn't.

You even want to track the quality and types of foods you eat.

Too often our belief that we "need carbs" leads to us eating a ton of processed junk food which can actually HINDER our performance long-term.

While there are lots of recovery aids and gels out there, we have to remember that quality does help our body function more efficiently!

Does Meal Timing Matter?

While the overall macro ratios and calories we hit for the day are most important, we can maximize our results and enhance our training by how we time our meals and especially our carbs.

Before a long run, make sure to get a good chunk of your carbs and fat, especially if your runs are hitting that 90 minute mark.

Post run, get a good deal of protein and carbs, but keep fat lower.

You can then consume the rest of your protein earlier and later in the day. But you want those carbs timed around your workouts to fuel your runs.

This isn't to say you can't train fasted IF you feel best that way.

If you are a morning exerciser, you may not only want to eat prior to your run or ride but also make sure your DINNER the night before is more carb heavy.

Adjusting your meal timing can really help you make sure you feel fueled without overeating or consuming more carbs than are actually needed.

Supplements For Endurance Athletes

So I know there are lots of carb supplements out there, but unless you are an elite runner or cyclist...well you probably don't need them if you dial in your nutrition properly.

Not to say you can't fit them in if they make you feel better, but make sure to log them so you can truly track.

An often overlooked supplement that can benefit endurance athletes is BCAAs.

Because steady-state cardio can be catabolic to muscle tissue, BCAAs can help prevent some muscle tissue breakdown AND even provide extra energy when consumed in your water during your run or ride.

Caffeine could be another way to "enhance" your performance. Consuming coffee or tea prior can enhance your performance for up to 6 hours. However, you do want to be careful with any stimulant.

Final Tips For Endurance Athletes

The one thing that is 100% certain is that you should NOT change anything only weeks before a race. At that point, you have to go with what you've been doing.

I recommend if you want to play around with your nutrition, that you start experimenting in your off season or around practice races. You want to have that routine dialed in when you are training to hit that PR!

Managing Hormones

Ok ladies...this section is for you!

Let's talk about hormones!

Because those female hormones will affect not only how you diet at certain times of the month, but also as you get older!

First...let's talk about that monthly "friend"...

Dieting Around Your Period

Guess what?!

You feel hungrier and get cravings before your period for a reason!

So instead of beating yourself up for your "slip ups" around that time of the month, and instead of fighting against the fact that you feel hungrier, why not try to work WITH your body!?

It's time we started adjusting our diets with our cycles so we don't feel like everything just goes out the window and we are constantly having to start over each month.

How can you deal with those cravings while staying on track since for some of us this is a monthly issue!?

STEP #1 - Adjust Calories

The first way you can handle your hunger is by increasing your calories. You get hungrier because your metabolic rate actually does increase!

Instead of fighting against the fact that you are hungrier, give yourself a calorie bump.

This can help you avoid binging and keep you on track. And because you are burning more calories even at rest, the calorie bump won't necessarily kick you out of a deficit if you are trying to lose weight.

This calorie bump can also allow you to fit in an extra treat or two so that you don't feel guilty about indulging.

Sometimes the fact that we've kept to our plan helps mentally, even if the quality of our food isn't "ideal." This balance is key for long-term adherence and lasting results!

You can adjust your calories up as PMS hits and the cravings start, and then adjust back down when you start menstruation and your metabolic rate slows back down.

Give yourself a range even, allowing 200-400 more calories on the days you feel hungrier. You can even decide to take a Diet Break around this time of the month.

Sometimes just knowing you CAN increase calories if needed helps even if you don't end up eating more.

STEP #2 - Don't Make Foods Off Limits

When cravings hit, while we don't always want to make an excuse to indulge, there are times we can't resist.

Better to not feel guilty for indulging, which will only lead to further binging.

Better to PLAN to allow these foods, even if you may decide to make them "off limits" at other times.

And if you know what you tend to crave, you can even plan ahead and find "healthier" options.

If you tend to crave chocolate, find a chocolate bar you can fit into your macros, maybe making it darker chocolate if you want to stay lower carb.

Or if you crave ice cream, maybe try a low calorie alternative or a greek yogurt homemade version.

So not only can you plan to indulge, but you can also plan in healthier versions of those foods you crave, which can help you stay on track.

The key is to not have foods be "off limits" around this time of the month, which often makes cravings even worse!

STEP #3 - Adjust Your Macros

Some women tend to crave carbs more. Others tend to crave fats more.

I have yet to have a woman tell me she craves protein, but if you do...go for it!

Whatever you find yourself wanting more of, plan to adjust your macros to allow for it. Pick a ratio that will be easier for you to stick to, even if you only do it for the week or just a couple of days!

This doesn't mean making 60% of your calories carbs and 30% fat just so you can fit in a ton of chocolate, but it does mean picking a ratio that allows you to respond to your cravings.

Often even just a more moderate ratio of 30% protein, 35% carbs, 35% fat can be good as it keeps you on track, BUT gives you more freedom.

Remember the worse thing we can do to ourselves is make ourselves feel guilty!

If something feels planned and "acceptable," we don't feel as guilty or bad for indulging, which makes it so much easier to stay on track overall and get consistent.

So plan around those cravings and adjust your macros!

STEP #4 - Be Prepared To Track And Adapt

Even when we plan ahead and give ourselve more flexibility, there will still be times we eat for emotional reasons.

It simply happens.

While you're always trying to work to have a healthier and better relationship with your body and with food, there are going to be those times we get mad or stressed or tired or whatever, and we end up binging.

We start and we can't stop.

And before we know it the whole pint of ice cream is gone.

The key is not making ourselves feel guilty about it.

If you "over indulge," don't feel like you've ruined the day.

Have the other healthy meals you've planned and just get right back "on track."

Depending on the indulgence too, often if you log it and track, you can "salvage" the day.

The key is just not believing that a day or week is "ruined" because you overindulged and gave into an unplanned craving.

Listen To Your Body

While we don't want to use our periods as an excuse to forget about our diet and binge eat everything in sight, we do want to recognize the changes that can occur.

We may even want to adjust our workouts as our periods can even impact our training routine.

And it's actually not all bad!

These hormone changes can work to your advantage.

Take advantage of the fact that you may actually burn more fat, and have a greater "after burn" effect from your workouts during the luteal phase, which is about 11-14 days prior to your next period.

This may also cause you to be hungrier so you might find slightly switching your meal timing to be key. You might want to include a post-workout snack even if you don't usually have one. If you already have a post-workout snack, you may want to add an extra 100-200 calories into that meal.

Dieting For Menopause

Even after we are done with monthly periods, those dang female hormones can still cause problems. It's almost not fair!

When our hormones change with menopause, it can be a struggle to keep the weight off.

And often the dieting practices we've followed in the past not only won't work, but may even be causing us to struggle to get the results we want.

Macros Matter!

Basically, increasing your protein intake is key. Hitting a minimum of 30% protein becomes more and more important and beneficial no matter where your fat and carb intakes fall.

As we get older, and our hormones change, it becomes more difficult to not only build lean muscle mass, but even retain the lean muscle mass we currently have.

The decline in estrogen that occurs with menopause has been linked to a decrease in muscle mass and even bone strength.

This is why not only strength training is so important, but also increasing our protein intake.

We become less efficient at protein synthesis so we need more protein to help repair and build muscle tissue.

Protein is also key to keeping our skin, hair and nails healthy and strong! It may be why women going through menopause benefit from a collagen supplement.

During, and even post-menopause, protein can help keep our hormones in check and help us avoid that dreaded weight gain that often occurs.

In menopause, your hormone levels change and even specific hormones decrease. So if you don't get enough protein, you're going to have a harder time maintaining hormonal balance, which can further negatively impact muscle retention and cause weight gain.

It can also affect our digestive system, thyroid and bone health! Getting more protein can help keep our bones strong to avoid hip fractures!

So while you may be looking to change up your diet to avoid gaining that dreaded belly fat, increasing your protein really is key for overall health.

So what macro ranges should you use?

Protein: Keep your protein intake at about 30%. While you can increase protein up to 50% if you're training hard and really want to focus on gaining muscle, 30% is enough to help you retain lean muscle mass even with the hormonal changes.

Carbs: As we get older, our metabolic rate naturally slows down some. Because of this, lowering your carb intake can help you prevent weight gain. A range of 20-30% carbs works well although endurance athletes, or those potentially even in a muscle gaining phase, may go higher.

Fat: "Healthy fats" especially omega-3s can have anti-inflammatory benefits, which becomes more and more key as we get older. Also, omega-3s have even been shown to potentially help with hot flashes and other menopause-related symptoms. So a diet higher in fat can be helpful. While you can drop your fat intake to 25%, generally keeping it between 30-40% works best. For those struggling to lose weight, even increasing fat intake to 50% may help.

What ratios should you start with?

Because "healthy" fats and protein are essential, and our overall resting energy expenditure decreases with age, generally a slightly higher fat and higher protein ratio is key.

If you do more endurance activities, you will still want to make sure you're getting enough carbs although 30% is often more than enough.

Below are 4 ratios that work well for avoiding muscle loss and weight gain during menopause:

-30% protein/30% carbs/40% fat
-45% protein/20% carbs/35% fat
-30% protein/20% carbs/50% fat
-40% protein/30% carbs/30% fat

How should you cycle the ratios?

If your goal is weight loss, cycle the ratios every 1-3 weeks, using these 3 breakdowns below:

Weeks 1-3: 30% protein/20% carbs/50% fat
Weeks 4-6: 40% protein/30% carbs/30% fat
Weeks 7-9: 45% protein/20% carbs/35% fat

If you want to build muscle, change ratios as you change your programming every 3-6 weeks.

However, if building muscle is your main focus, you may also want to add in a higher carb ratio to your cycle from the Muscle Macros section with these two ratios:

Weeks 1-3: 30% protein/30% carbs/40% fat
Weeks 4-6: Muscle Building Higher Carb Breakdown
Weeks 7-9: 40% protein/30% carbs/30% fat.

If you want to focus on maintaining your current weight, while potentially shedding just a little bit of fat, cycle the ratios every 1-4 weeks. You may also want to stick with these 3 ratios:

Weeks 1-2: 30% protein/30% carbs/40% fat
Weeks 3-4: 45% protein/20% carbs/35% fat
Weeks 5-6: 40% protein/30% carbs/30% fat

How Many Calories Do You Need?

One of the dieting practices that holds us back the most as we go through menopause is our belief that we need to create as big a deficit as possible.

But cutting your calories too low may be causing you to gain weight.

We already struggle to retain lean muscle mass and avoid our metabolism "slowing down" as we get older.

We only make that cycle worse if we don't eat enough.

So even if you want to lose weight, start with a calorie intake no lower than 11x goal bodyweight.

If you've been consuming well below this intake, slowly bump up your calories by 100-200 until you reach that number. You will want to adjust slowly over a couple of weeks to help your body "learn" to eat more.

If you want to build muscle, you may start your intake at 13-14x goal bodyweight (which may be your current bodyweight).

Do not fear more calories though, even when trying to lose weight, as we need to eat enough to promote optimal hormone levels and avoid muscle catabolism!

Should Our Diet Change As We Get Older?

While women will want to adjust their diets because of menopause, ALL of us need to be conscious of the impact that getting older has on our body and our nutritional needs.

The more we recognize the changes our body goes through as we get older, the better we can tailor our diet to meet our needs so we can get better results faster!

So what changes can occur as we get older?

As we get older we may notice a few changes occurring:

-Our metabolism slows down
-We may not tolerate certain foods, or alcohol, as well
-We may struggle to put on muscle and retain muscle as easily
-We may not lose fat as easily.
-We may take longer to recover from intense workouts
But these changes don't have to hold us back from reaching our goals or feeling healthy and energized at every age!

Does Your Metabolism ACTUALLY Slow Down? And If So, Why!?

As we get older, our metabolism does slow down.

If you don't have as much muscle mass, you aren't going to burn as many calories at rest.

And this problem is only made worse by the fact that we become less active as we get older.

Because we are less active, we aren't expending as much energy in general throughout the day.

We also have a tendency to not train as hard, which means we aren't promoting muscle growth.

This can cause our body composition to become worse as we get older age, which will only further lower our metabolic rate.

So while yes, your metabolism will slow down, we can prevent some of that adaptation by staying active!

We may not be able to control our age, but we can still workout hard and dial in our diet to promote better muscle retention!

Because the more muscle mass we have, the higher our metabolic rate will be!

And keeping our metabolism "healthy" may be the key to living longer!

A study showed that a key to longevity may be avoiding the metabolic slow down often associated with old age.

So don't just accept that your metabolism is going to slow down! Do what you can to prevent it!

Why Protein Is Essential As We Get Older

As we get older, our body becomes less efficient at utilizing protein.

Since we have lower rates of protein synthesis, we have more trouble gaining, let alone retaining, lean muscle mass.

The loss of lean muscle mass can lower our metabolic rate.

So increasing our protein is key to helping us maintain our lean muscle mass.

And protein also has the added benefit of a higher thermic effect than carbs or fat.

This means that eating a higher protein diet can actually boost your metabolism and help you burn more calories without even changing your activity level.

Anything we can do to boost our metabolic rate can help us avoid the dreaded weight gain often associated with getting older.

As we get older too, it can take us longer to recover from intense training sessions.

Increasing our protein intake, can also help improve our recovery so we can continue to train hard and even compete.

You may want to even consider a BCAA supplement to help you recover faster, especially if you're training hard or struggling to increase your protein intake.

Leucine, found in BCAAs, is thought to offer the greatest benefit when it comes to preserving muscle mass and function as we get older.

Even increasing the protein you consume immediately post workout can help promote muscle growth and retention as well as improve your recovery.

Studies have shown that we may need to eat double the protein post workout as we get older to help us recover.

So even adjusting your meal timing can help!

Two other supplements to consider are collagen and creatine.

Collagen can help improve our recovery, protect our joints and even keep our skin, hair and nails healthy!

Creatine can help prevent the loss of bone density and muscle mass. It can also help improve your workouts by preventing fatigue and improving your strength, power and work capacity.

This means you can train harder which can result in better muscle growth and even fat loss!

What Ratios Should You Use?

Focus on increasing your protein intake to at least 30% of your calories to start.

If you are training hard, and want to gain muscle and even lose fat, consider a higher protein ratio such as 40-50%.

Depending on your training routine, you can adjust carbs and fat as needed. And, if you're going through menopause, you'll want to check out the Managing Hormones ratios.

If you're looking to remain active and stay lean, these 6 breakdowns are a great place to start:

-40% protein/30% carbs/30% fat
-45% protein/35% carbs/20% fat
-45% protein/20% carbs/35% fat
-30% protein/30% carbs/40% fat
-50% protein/30% carbs/20% fat
-30% protein/40% carbs/30% fat

You will want to cycle these ratios every 3-4 weeks, or with changes to your workout routine.
If your goal is fat loss, cycling every 2 weeks works best!

How Many Calories Do You Need?

Eating in a bigger calorie deficit won't speed up your results. As you get older, it may end up holding you back more and more.

You may actually be better off first adjusting your macros without adjusting your calorie intake because we need to eat enough calories to promote not only muscle retention but even potentially muscle growth!

If you're training hard and not eating enough, you may actually end up causing more damage. You may end up catabolizing your muscle mass in order to provide your body with the fuel it needs!

Plus, extreme calorie restriction causes our body to conserve energy and our metabolism slows in response.

So make sure that even if you are trying to create a calorie deficit, you start with no lower than 11x goal bodyweight (which may be your current bodyweight).

If you are training intensely, set your calorie intake at even 13-14x goal bodyweight.

As we get older, our appetite can also sometimes change. We may not feel as hungry, which can make it challenging to eat more. So changing up our meal frequency may help.

Supplements and smaller, more frequent meals may help us eat enough while still hitting our macro ratios.

Where Do You Start!?

Develop proper eating habits as early on as possible!

And remember, it is never too late to make changes!

Work to find a balance you can maintain - not just a quick fix.

Know there will be ups and downs. Times you "cut" and times you "bulk." But work to make those cycles smaller.

When we've spent years going from extreme diet to extreme diet, we've often caused our body composition to become worse and worse, which only contributes to our struggles as we get older.

We decrease our calories so significantly that our body preserves fat stores. Because insulin is low, our thyroid hormone production decreases.

Then, because of this, our resting metabolism is lowered.

And this can take place within just 24 hours of starting an extreme diet!!

Because of our body's response to calorie deprivation, we often rebound and gain all of the weight, and even more!, back once we fall off the diet because it isn't sustainable.

We lose muscle mass in our attempts to lose weight fast and end up with larger fat stores.

Less lean muscle mass, results in a lowered metabolic rate.

This then fights against us the next time we try to diet down.

So while it can be so tempting to try something that promises faster results, remember that you want lasting results as well!

It all boils down to macros and creating the calorie intake right for your goals!

And then, don't be afraid to track and adapt your diet over time!

Now What About Alcohol?

To drink or not to drink...that is the question…

But it really isn't a question of should you drink, but rather are you going to drink?

Because the simple fact is...If you're asking about alcohol now, chances are you want an excuse to include it.

And even if I tell you not to drink, you're going to anyway.

You may be able to restrict your alcohol intake for a bit, but if you're asking about whether or not you can include it, it's probably going to creep back in because it's a part of your lifestyle that you enjoy.

Realistically, you're not going to cut it out long term. So maybe you shouldn't ever even force that change.

Now note, this is of course a discussion about "healthy" overall alcohol intake and a "healthy" relationship to drinking so if discussing alcohol is a trigger, please ignore this section and know I will love you for doing so.

But if you choose to include alcohol, there's one thing I'll tell you right now…

No alcohol is healthy.

Now don't go trying to defend the health benefits of your wine…Cause that just really isn't all that it's touted to be.

First off, most of us DO NOT actually get those supposed benefits.

And secondly, most of us aren't really consuming wine for its health benefits (And we aren't consuming it in the EXTREMELY moderate amounts it should be consumed.)

We drink alcohol because we like it and enjoy the social gatherings that often come with it.

And there is nothing wrong with that. But we can't lie to ourselves about it being "healthy."

Because basically studies show that the healthiest amount of alcohol is ZERO.

Sorry to break it to you, but as I jokingly say all of the time – Alcohol is a toxin.

There really no health benefits that outweigh the risks.

But that doesn't mean there can't be a reason to ENJOY alcohol.

I would argue the only real "benefit" of alcohol is that you ENJOY it and life is meant to be enjoyed.

And that by relaxing, and enjoying a couple of drinks with friends, you can lower stress levels, which may, in the end, do much more to benefit your overall health than a few drinks will do to negatively impact it.

Because STRESS does play a major role in our overall health. Much more of one than we give it credit for.

So if alcohol is a part of your lifestyle, it doesn't have to be eliminated.

I do recommend though, when you're first starting out, to keep it to your "cheat day" or at least 1-2 set days a week.

Alcohol won't promote better results and may actually SLOW your results regardless of your goal.

But, it can be part of your lifestyle balance.

So...How do you TRACK alcohol if you're counting macros?

Logging alcohol is an interesting thing.

While beer and wine will register a few carbs, alcohol will register as calories but not really a macro since it's… well…it's own macro.

So if you're trying to track and log, you can count it as either a fat or carb. I recommend counting it as whichever you have more of with the ratio you are using.

You will then divide the calories in your alcohol by 4 for carbs or 9 for fat to get the total grams of each you would have consumed. (No you can't count it as protein!)

If you can, I do recommend counting alcohol as a fat because alcohol suppresses fat oxidation.

While alcohol can fit into a balanced lifestyle, even while you're tracking to get a specific result, if you want FASTER RESULTS, eliminating alcohol, if even just for a time, can be key.

Alcohol can slow our results by negatively impacting our training sessions, even the sessions done prior to our night out drinking.

Consuming alcohol after our training session can inhibit protein synthesis and lipolysis (or fat loss).

So if you're looking to gain muscle or lose fat, frequent alcohol consumption will work against your results no matter how well you eat or how precisely you hit your macros.

Not to mention it usually makes for a crappier training session the next day!

For men, alcohol also has a bigger impact on testosterone levels, which can further impact the gains you work so hard to create in the gym.

And alcohol can also perpetuate and create inflammation, which can not only make you feel aches and pains from your workouts more but be detrimental to your recovery!

Basically, alcohol fights against all of your hard work and can make it take that much longer to get the results you really want.

And not only does the alcohol itself negatively impact our bodies, but...let's face it…most of us also end up making poor food choices if we've had a few too many drinks.

So, while I'm sure this sounded negative, you can find a balance and include alcohol, you just need to make sure to track and recognize that faster results may mean eliminating it for a bit until you're in more of a maintenance phase!

Just go in with your eyes wide open when you do decide to indulge!

Implementing Your Diet Plan

You've calculated your calorie intake. You've set your macros.

Now comes the hardest part…

Actually getting started!

While this change can seem scary, you're ready for it. And there is no time like the present to get started.

Here are 3 final tips to help you get started today and make your diet change a huge success!

1. **Set an end date**
2. **Don't judge**
3. **Commit to a plan no matter what**

#1: Set An End Date

We want to create habit changes that build a new lifestyle. But the idea of doing something forever, of having no end date, is intimidating.

So even if you want to make lasting changes, break down your plan into cycles with specific end dates.

It's why committing to one of the 4-9 week cycles I have in this guide can be key.

When we have an end date in sight, we are far more motivated to get started immediately and stick with the plan.

An end date can provide some accountability and even "pressure" to stay committed.

It also gives a point at which we can assess our progress and make changes. This can prevent us from jumping ship too soon.

Sometimes if we don't have an end date and then "feel" like we aren't making progress, we give up.

Why continue on and risk wasting more time?

But when we have an end date it can be easier to see all of it as experiment and ride out the ups and downs.

Because no matter what, we have a point at which we can make a change.

So set an end date and even mark that date on your calendar with something fun to celebrate it and keep you motivated and moving forward!

#2: Don't Judge

We are our own harshest critics most of the time. We eat one thing "off plan" and act like the whole thing is ruined.

We force ourselves to "start over" because we ruined a day.

Stop judging yourself.

There will be ups and downs. Mistakes and set backs.

But what makes these "slip ups" result in complete failures isn't the mistake itself, but our attitude toward it.

When you get started tracking, pretend you are your own teacher.

Talk to yourself like you would a student learning a new subject.

Because if you treat yourself like you would a student, you'll probably be a whole heck of a lot nicer and less judgmental.

You'll realize that it isn't about perfection, but about consistency and hard work day in and day out.

And the less you judge?

The more likely you are to succeed because there won't be the pressure to be perfect!

#3: Commit To A Plan No Matter What

We are human. There are going to be ups and downs. And we need to stick with our plan through those good and bad phases.

And not only that, but we have to remember that results take time to add up.

There are going to be periods where you feel like you aren't making progress at all. It's called the "dead zone" and occurs most often with fat loss diets.

During this time you can not only feel like nothing is happening, but that you're actually going backward.

And because we feel like nothing is happening, we give up.

Too often we stop right before we would have hit the jackpot.

Often we quit right before those results start snowballing.

You may not see the changes right away, but if you're tracking and logging and following the plan, you need to trust the process, knowing that things are happening!

Momentum, results, take time to build.

So decide upon a plan and see it through! You may be surprised by how those results finally add up right after when you would have usually given up!

One Final Thought - If You Have A Question Ask!

One last final thought...if, at any time, you need help, don't hesitate to reach out.

The only dumb question is the one you have and don't ask!

MACRO {HACKS}

MEAL GUIDES

Meal Guides Table of Contents

Meal Plan
TRADITIONAL: 30P/40C/30F

1300 Calories	1500 Calories	1700 Calories
Daily Macros	**Daily Macros**	**Daily Macros**
Calories: 1306 Protein: 110g Carbs: 129g Fat: 40g	Calories: 1525 Protein: 121g Carbs: 154g Fat: 52g	Calories: 1717 Protein: 139g Carbs: 170g Fat: 59g
Breakfast	**Breakfast**	**Breakfast**
Sweet Potato Egg Nest	Sweet Potato Egg Nest	Sweet Potato Egg Nest 1/2 cup Nonfat Greek Yogurt 1/2 cup Blueberries
Snack	**Snack**	**Snack**
1 cup Raspberries 2/3 oz Almonds	1 1/2 cup Raspberries 1 oz Almonds 1 Hard Boiled Egg	1 1/2 cup Raspberries 1 oz Almonds 1 Hard Boiled Egg
Lunch	**Lunch**	**Lunch**
Easy Crockpot Chili	Easy Crockpot Chili	Easy Crockpot Chili
Snack	**Snack**	**Snack**
Homemade Tortilla Chips 1/4 cup Salsa	Homemade Tortilla Chips 1/4 cup Salsa 1 1/2 cup Cherry Tomatoes	Homemade Tortilla Chips 1/4 cup Salsa 1 1/2 cup Cherry Tomatoes 1 Cheddar Cheese Stick
Dinner	**Dinner**	**Dinner**
Sheet Pan Chicken & Asparagus	Sheet Pan Chicken & Asparagus	Sheet Pan Chicken & Asparagus

Sweet Potato Egg Nests

SERVINGS	CALORIES	MACROS
3	260	P: 15g C: 29g F: 10g

INGREDIENTS

1/4 cup Diced Onion
1/2 cup Bell Pepper (any color)
6 Large Eggs
2 Large Sweet Potatoes

INSTRUCTIONS

***NOTE: Makes 6 servings or 2 nests per serving

Preheat the oven to 400F.

Using a cheese grater, grate the sweet potato into little shreds.

Spray a muffin tin with nonstick spray, then add the sweet potato shreds into the cups and mold them into little nests (pushing against the bottom and sides of the cup).

Bake them for 15 minutes.

Dice onion and bell pepper.

Remove the nests from the oven, add the diced veggies to the nests and crack an egg into each. Sprinkle with salt and pepper if desired.

Bake for an additional 12 minutes, 15 minutes if you want harder yolks.

Easy Crockpot Chili

SERVINGS	CALORIES	MACROS
3	410	P: 34g C: 48g F: 9g

INGREDIENTS

2/3 pound 93% Ground Turkey
8 oz Corn, Kernels
15 oz Red Kidney Beans
14 1/2 oz Tomato Sauce
14 1/2 oz Diced Tomatoes
2 cups Water

INSTRUCTIONS

In a nonstick skillet, turkey beef until no longer pink.

Add all ingredients to a crockpot. Add any spices if you choose.

Cook on LOW for 6-7 hours or HIGH for 4 hours.

Homemade Tortilla Chips

SERVINGS	CALORIES	MACROS
1	100	P: 3g C: 20g F: 1.5g

INGREDIENTS

2 Corn Tortillas

INSTRUCTIONS

Preheat oven to 350F.

Spray a cookie sheet with nonstick cooking spray.

Cut each tortilla into chip sized wedges and arrange the wedges in a single layer on a cookie sheet.

Bake for about 7 minutes. Flip the chips and bake for another 8 minutes or until the chips are crisp, but not too brown. Make sure not to burn!

Sheet Pan Chicken & Asparagus

SERVINGS	CALORIES	MACROS
3	330	P: 52g C: 8g F: 10g

INGREDIENTS

1 tbsp Olive Oil
2 tbsp Lemon Juice
3 Garlic Cloves
1 tsp Dried Parsley
1/2 tsp Dried Rosemary
1 pound Chicken Breast (boneless, skinless)
1 pound Fresh Asparagus

INSTRUCTIONS

***Also Needed: Parchment Paper

Preheat oven to 425F.

In a small bowl, mix olive oil, lemon juice, garlic, parsley and rosemary together.

Add chicken to a parchment-lined baking sheet and toss with lemon mixture. Add salt and pepper if desired. Bake for 15 minutes.

Meanwhile, trim ends of asparagus. When chicken is cooked for approximately 15 minutes, add asparagus to the pan and bake for 8-10 minutes until tender and chicken is cooked through.

Meal Plan
TRADITIONAL: 40P/30C/30F

1300 Calories	1500 Calories	1700 Calories
Daily Macros	**Daily Macros**	**Daily Macros**
Calories: 1319	Calories: 1514	Calories: 1697
Protein: 151g	Protein: 158g	Protein: 176g
Carbs: 95g	Carbs: 117g	Carbs: 130g
Fat: 41g	Fat: 52g	Fat: 59g
Breakfast	**Breakfast**	**Breakfast**
Skinny Ham & Cheese Frittata	Skinny Ham & Cheese Frittata	Skinny Ham & Cheese Frittata
		1/2 cup Nonfat Cottage Cheese
Snack	**Snack**	**Snack**
1 Banana	1 Banana	1 Banana
1 1/2 tbsp Peanut Butter	3 tbsp Peanut Butter	3 tbsp Peanut Butter
Lunch	**Lunch**	**Lunch**
Easy Kung Pao Chicken	Easy Kung Pao Chicken	Easy Kung Pao Chicken
1 cup Cauliflower Rice	1 cup Cauliflower Rice	1 cup Cauliflower Rice
Snack	**Snack**	**Snack**
1 cup Cherry Tomatoes	2 cup Cherry Tomatoes	2 cup Cherry Tomatoes
Protein Shake -	Protein Shake -	Protein Shake -
30 grams Protein Powder	30 grams Protein Powder	30 grams Protein Powder
		1/2 oz Almonds
Dinner	**Dinner**	**Dinner**
Turkey Skillet with Veggies	Turkey Skillet with Veggies	Turkey Skillet with Veggies
2 oz Green Beans	4 oz Green Beans	6 oz Green Beans

Skinny Ham & Cheese Frittata

SERVINGS	CALORIES	MACROS
3	220	P: 33g C: 7g F: 6g

INGREDIENTS

1 cup Extra Lean Ham
1/4 tsp Cayenne Pepper
1 1/2 cups Egg Whites
1/4 cup Mozzarella Cheese (shredded, reduced fat)
1/2 tsp Garlic Powder
2 cups Spinach
1 cup Cherry Tomatoes
1/4 cup Diced Onion
1/3 cup Sliced Mushrooms

INSTRUCTIONS

Preheat your oven to 400F.

In a medium bowl, whisk egg whites, garlic powder and cayenne pepper. Add salt and black pepper if desired.

Add shredded cheese and gently stir to combine.

In a nonstick skillet, cook onions over medium heat until tender (about 2 minutes).

Pour egg white mixture into skillet.

Place chopped vegetables and ham into egg white mixture.

Cook for about 2-3 minutes on medium heat on the stove top, or until edges of frittata are set.

Remove from stove top and transfer to your preheated oven to cook for an additional 3-4 minutes, or until egg whites are set and cooked.

Easy Kung Pao Chicken

SERVINGS	CALORIES	MACROS
3	360	P: 50g C: 17g F: 10g

INGREDIENTS

2 tsp Sriracha
1 tbsp Honey
1/4 cup Coconut Aminos
1 pound Chicken Breast (boneless, skinless)
1 tbsp Sesame Oil
3 Garlic Raw Cloves
2 tsp Minced Ginger
1 Bell Pepper (any color)
3 cups Broccoli Florets

INSTRUCTIONS

Combine all sauce ingredients in a bowl (coconut aminos, honey and sriracha).

Heat 1/2 tbsp sesame oil in a large sauté pan or wok.

Once hot, add chicken, garlic and ginger and cook for 5-7 minutes until chicken is just cooked through. Transfer chicken to a plate.

In the same pan, add remaining oil, bell pepper and broccoli; mix well. Cook for 5 minutes or until broccoli is tender, then add chicken and sauce to the pan and cook for 2-3 minutes or until sauce thickens a bit.

Turn off heat and let rest for 2-3 minutes.

Turkey Skillet with Veggies

SERVINGS	CALORIES	MACROS
3	280	P: 32g C: 14g F: 11g

INGREDIENTS

1 pound 93% Ground Turkey
2 Zucchini
3 grams Garlic Clove
1/2 cup Diced Onion
1 cup Diced Bell Pepper (any color)
3/4 cup Tomato Sauce

INSTRUCTIONS

In a nonstick skillet, over medium-high heat, add ground turkey and break it up until it's in small pieces.

Once the turkey is almost cooked through, add the diced onion and garlic. Stir occasionally and cook until onions are golden brown.

Add diced bell peppers (you can use any color), chopped zucchini and tomato sauce.

Cover the skillet and cook until they are tender.

Add salt, black pepper, and crushed red pepper to taste if desired.

Meal Plan
TRADITIONAL: 30P/20C/50F

1300 Calories	1500 Calories	1700 Calories
Daily Macros	**Daily Macros**	**Daily Macros**
Calories: 1310	Calories: 1511	Calories: 1700
Protein: 109g	Protein: 120g	Protein: 127g
Carbs: 66g	Carbs: 80g	Carbs: 101g
Fat: 72g	Fat: 85g	Fat: 96g
Breakfast	**Breakfast**	**Breakfast**
Broccoli and Cheese Egg Cups	Broccoli and Cheese Egg Cups	Broccoli and Cheese Egg Cups
	1 cup Cherry Tomatoes	2 cups Cherry Tomatoes
Snack	**Snack**	**Snack**
3/4 oz Almonds	1 oz Almonds	1 1/2 oz Almonds
1 Hard Boiled Egg	2 Hard Boiled Eggs	2 Hard Boiled Eggs
Lunch	**Lunch**	**Lunch**
Baked Salmon in Foil	Baked Salmon in Foil	Baked Salmon in Foil
1/4 cup Cooked Quinoa	1/4 cup Cooked Quinoa	1/4 cup Cooked Quinoa
5 oz Green Beans	5 oz Green Beans	7 oz Green Beans
Snack	**Snack**	**Snack**
2 tbsp Peanut Butter	2 1/2 tbsp Peanut Butter	3 tbsp Peanut Butter
2 Celery Stalk	2 Celery Stalk	3 Celery Stalk
1 cup Raspberries	1 cup Raspberries	1 cup Raspberries
Dinner	**Dinner**	**Dinner**
Baked Pork Chops	Baked Pork Chops	Baked Pork Chops
1 Zucchini	1 Zucchini	1 Zucchini

Broccoli and Cheese Egg Cups

SERVINGS	CALORIES	MACROS
6	170	P: 14g C: 3g F: 13g

INGREDIENTS

10 Large Eggs
1/2 tsp Salt
1/2 tsp Ground Black Pepper
1/2 tsp Dried Thyme
1/2 tsp Garlic Powder
1 1/2 cups Broccoli Florets
2/3 cup Cheddar Cheese, Shredded

INSTRUCTIONS

***NOTE: Each serving is 2 cups

Preheat oven to 400F.

Line a 12 count muffin pan with silicone liners or coat with non-stick cooking spray. Set aside.

In a large bowl, crack in eggs and whisk together with salt and black pepper.

Whisk in garlic powder and thyme until combined. Stir in broccoli and cheddar.

Divide evenly into muffin tins.

Bake in preheated oven for 12-15 minutes, or until set.

Baked Salmon in Foil

SERVINGS	CALORIES	MACROS
3	260	P: 36g C: 2g F: 12g

INGREDIENTS

1 Lemon
1 pound Salmon
1 tbsp Olive Oil
3 Garlic Cloves

INSTRUCTIONS

Preheat the oven to 375F.

Slice the lemons and lay them down on a cookie sheet. Place the salmon on top and top with olive oil. Sprinkle with salt and pepper; scatter minced garlic. Bake the salmon for 20-25 minutes, until the salmon is completely cooked through at the thickest part.

Baked Pork Chops

SERVINGS	CALORIES	MACROS
3	270	P: 32g C: 2g F: 14g

INGREDIENTS

1 tbsp Ground Paprika
2 tsp Onion Powder
2 tsp Garlic Powder
1 tsp Ground Black Pepper
1 tsp Salt
1 tbsp Olive Oil 1 Tbsp
1 pound Pork Chops (Top Loin, Boneless)

INSTRUCTIONS

Preheat oven to 400F.

In a small bowl, mix together the paprika, onion powder, garlic powder, salt, pepper and oregano.

Drizzle the olive oil over both sides of the pork chops. Sprinkle the spice mix evenly over both sides of the pork chops and place them in a baking dish.

Bake the pork chops for approximately 18 minutes. Once you remove them from the oven, let them rest in the pan for 5 minutes before dividing.

Meal Plan
TRADITIONAL: 45P/30C/25F

1300 Calories	1500 Calories	1700 Calories
Daily Macros	**Daily Macros**	**Daily Macros**
Calories: 1310 Protein: 142g Carbs: 99g Fat: 36g	Calories: 1497 Protein: 166g Carbs: 116g Fat: 40g	Calories: 1696 Protein: 185g Carbs: 130g Fat: 49g
Breakfast	**Breakfast**	**Breakfast**
Cinnamon Quinoa Bowl	Cinnamon Quinoa Bowl 56 grams Turkey Bacon	Cinnamon Quinoa Bowl 84 grams Turkey Bacon
Snack	**Snack**	**Snack**
1/2 cup Nonfat Greek Yogurt 30 grams Optimum Nutrition Protein Powder 1/4 cup Blueberries	1 cup Nonfat Greek Yogurt 30 grams Optimum Nutrition Protein Powder 1/3 cup Blueberries	1 1/3 cup Nonfat Greek Yogurt 30 grams Optimum Nutrition Protein Powder 1/3 cup Blueberries
Lunch	**Lunch**	**Lunch**
Orange Chicken & Broccoli	Orange Chicken & Broccoli	Orange Chicken & Broccoli
Snack	**Snack**	**Snack**
1 oz Almonds 1 Cheddar Cheese Stick	1 oz Almonds 1 Cheddar Cheese Stick 1 cup Strawberries	1 1/2 oz Almonds 1 Cheddar Cheese Stick 1 cup Strawberries
Dinner	**Dinner**	**Dinner**
Simple Meatloaf 4 oz Green Beans	Simple Meatloaf 4 oz Green Beans	Simple Meatloaf 8 oz Green Beans

Cinnamon Quinoa Bowl

SERVINGS	CALORIES	MACROS
2	190	P: 7g C: 31g F: 4g

INGREDIENTS

1/2 cup Strawberries
1/2 cup Quinoa, Uncooked
1 cup Plain Almond Milk, Unsweetened
2 Cinnamon Sticks
1/2 tsp Vanilla Extract

INSTRUCTIONS

Rinse and drain the quinoa.

Place it in a small saucepan and add the almond milk, 1-2 cinnamon sticks, vanilla, and a pinch of salt.

Bring to a high simmer, cover and reduce heat to a low simmer for 15 minutes. (Tip: don't walk away, if it starts bubbling, turn the heat off, give it one stir mid-cook if you need to, and resume).

After 15 minutes, remove the pan from the heat and let the quinoa sit for 5 more minutes or until the almond milk is absorbed and the quinoa is cooked. Taste and add additional spices to your liking.

Add the strawberries when ready to eat.

Orange Chicken and Broccoli

SERVINGS	CALORIES	MACROS
3	380	P: 49g C: 27g F: 8g

INGREDIENTS

1/2 tbsp Olive Oil
1 pound Chicken Breast (Boneless, Skinless)
1/4 cup Honey
2 tbsp Orange Juice
1/4 tsp Red Pepper Flakes
1/2 inch Fresh Ginger
1/4 tsp Ground Black Pepper
1 pound Broccoli Florets
3 Garlic Cloves

INSTRUCTIONS

Preheat oven to 400F.

Spread the broccoli out to the edges of a nonstick baking tray.

In a small bowl, whisk together honey, orange juice, olive oil, ginger, garlic cloves, red pepper flakes and black pepper.

Line chicken in the center of the pan. Season with salt, pepper and garlic powder as desired. Spread marinade evenly over chicken.

Place in oven and bake for about 20 minutes.

When you pull out the pan, some extra liquid will most likely be on it. Blot it with a paper towel or pour it gently off the side.

Simple Meatloaf

SERVINGS	CALORIES	MACROS
3	250	P: 37g C: 15g F: 2g

INGREDIENTS

1 pound 99% Lean Ground Turkey
1 Large Egg
1/2 cup Skim Milk
1/2 cup Panko Breadcrumbs
1/4 cup Diced Onion
1 tbsp Ketchup
1/2 tsp Italian Seasoning

INSTRUCTIONS

Preheat oven to 350F.

In a medium bowl combine the egg, milk and breadcrumbs. Allow mixture to sit for 5-10 minutes.

Then, add the ground turkey, onions and Italian seasoning. Mix until just combined.

Place mixture into a nonstick baking loaf and bake for approximately 50-60 minutes.

Allow meatloaf to rest for 10 minutes before slicing.

Meal Plan
TRADITIONAL: 35P/32C/33F

1300 Calories	1500 Calories	1700 Calories
Daily Macros	**Daily Macros**	**Daily Macros**
Calories: 1284 Protein: 117g Carbs: 105g Fat: 45g	Calories: 1492 Protein: 126g Carbs: 124g Fat: 56g	Calories: 1710 Protein: 151g Carbs: 139g Fat: 63g
Breakfast	**Breakfast**	**Breakfast**
Healthy Breakfast Casserole	Healthy Breakfast Casserole	Healthy Breakfast Casserole 2/3 cup Nonfat Cottage Cheese
Snack	**Snack**	**Snack**
1/3 cup Original Hummus 1/2 cup Baby Carrots	1/2 cup Original Hummus 2/3 cup Baby Carrots	1/2 cup Original Hummus 1 cup Baby Carrots
Lunch	**Lunch**	**Lunch**
Sheet Pan Chicken Fajitas 1/2 cup Cauliflower Rice	Sheet Pan Chicken Fajitas 1/2 cup Cauliflower Rice	Sheet Pan Chicken Fajitas 1/2 cup Cauliflower Rice
Snack	**Snack**	**Snack**
1 Hard Boiled Egg 2/3 cup Grapes	2 Hard Boiled Eggs 1 cup Grapes	2 Hard Boiled Eggs 1 cup Grapes 1 Cheddar Cheese Stick
Dinner	**Dinner**	**Dinner**
Asian Flank Steak 4 oz Sweet Potato	Asian Flank Steak 4 oz Sweet Potato	Asian Flank Steak 4 oz Sweet Potato

Healthy Breakfast Casserole

SERVINGS	CALORIES	MACROS
6	170	P: 18g C: 10g F: 6g

INGREDIENTS

1 Large Sweet Potato
2 cups Baby Spinach
1/3 cup Diced Onion
1 Green Bell Pepper
3 Garlic Cloves
112 grams Turkey Bacon
1 1/2 cups Egg Whites
6 Large Eggs
1/2 cup Plain Almond Milk, Unsweetened
1 tsp Ground Paprika

INSTRUCTIONS

Preheat oven to 350F.

Cook bacon in a nonstick pan.

Grate sweet potato and place into a nonstick casserole dish.

Add diced onion, bell pepper, garlic, and cooked bacon to the casserole dish. Mix all vegetables and bacon together. Set aside.

In a large bowl, whisk eggs and egg whites together until combined. Add milk and to the eggs and whisk again.

Next, add paprika, a pinch of salt, to egg mixture and whisk one final time.

Pour egg mixture into the casserole dish. Making sure all vegetables and bacon are covered. Mix in the spinach.

Place casserole dish into the oven and bake for approximately 35 minutes.

Sheet Pan Chicken Fajitas

SERVINGS	CALORIES	MACROS
3	290	P: 49g C: 12g F: 6g

INGREDIENTS

1 Lime
1/2 tsp Garlic Powder
1/2 tsp Ground Cumin
1 tsp Chili Powder
3 Bell Peppers (Any Color)
1/2 Onion
1 pound Chicken Breast (Boneless, Skinless)

INSTRUCTIONS

Preheat oven to 400F.

Dice the veggies and spread the peppers and onions evenly across the a nonstick baking sheet. Place in the oven and bake for 8 minutes.

Meanwhile, in the same bowl, combine the chicken, chili powder, cumin, garlic powder, salt and black pepper if desired.

Remove the sheet from the oven, drain off any excess liquid from the veggies and add the chicken.

Return to the oven and bake for 15-20 minutes or until the vegetables are roasted and the chicken is golden brown and cooked through.

Remove, squeeze the lime juice over top.

Asian Flank Steak

SERVINGS	CALORIES	MACROS
3	360	P: 33g C: 18g F: 16g

INGREDIENTS

1 tbsp Olive Oil
1/3 cup Coconut Aminos
2 tbsp Honey
3 Garlic Cloves
2 tbsp Fresh Rosemary
1 tbsp Balsamic Vinegar
1 pound Beef, Flank Steak

INSTRUCTIONS

***NOTE: Steak needs to marinate overnight.
****Also Needed: Ziploc Bag

Whisk all ingredients together in a bowl.

Place steak in a Ziploc Bag and pour marinade in. Place in refrigerator and let marinade overnight.

When you're ready to cook the steak remove it from the marinade.

Cook steak on a grill or in a skillet over medium-high heat for about 3-4 minutes per side.

Place on a cutting board to rest for about 10 minutes and then slice against the grain.

Meal Plan
TRADITIONAL/PALEO: 50P/30C/20F

1300 Calories	1500 Calories	1700 Calories
Daily Macros	**Daily Macros**	**Daily Macros**
Calories: 1301 Protein: 169g Carbs: 103g Fat: 31g	Calories: 1503 Protein: 193g Carbs: 114g Fat: 40g	Calories: 1691 Protein: 211g Carbs: 134g Fat: 44g
Breakfast	**Breakfast**	**Breakfast**
Green Smoothie	Green Smoothie	Green Smoothie
Snack	**Snack**	**Snack**
5 oz Tuna 1 cup Baby Carrots	5 oz Tuna 1 cup Baby Carrots 1/2 oz Cashews	6 1/2 oz Tuna 1 cup Baby Carrots 1/3 oz Cashews 1 Hard Boiled Egg
Lunch	**Lunch**	**Lunch**
Chicken and Broccoli Bowls	Chicken and Broccoli Bowls	Chicken and Broccoli Bowls 1 1/3 cup Strawberries
Snack	**Snack**	**Snack**
Zucchini Chips 1/3 cup Salsa 3 Celery Stalks	Zucchini Chips 1/3 cup Salsa 3 Celery Stalks Protein Shake - 30 grams Protein Powder	Zucchini Chips 1/2 cup Salsa 5 Celery Stalks Protein Shake - 30 grams Protein Powder
Dinner	**Dinner**	**Dinner**
Thai Turkey Burgers 8 oz Asparagus	Thai Turkey Burgers 10 oz Asparagus	Thai Turkey Burgers 10 oz Asparagus

Green Smoothie

SERVINGS	CALORIES	MACROS
1	340	P: 37g C: 35g F: 7g

INGREDIENTS

41 grams Vega Sport Performance Protein
1/2 cup Plain Almond Milk, Unsweetened
1 cup Kale
2 cups Baby Spinach
1/2 Banana
1/2 cup Strawberries
1/2 tbsp Chia Seeds

INSTRUCTIONS

Place everything in a blender and combine. Add more ice to reach a thicker consistency if desired.

Zucchini Chips

SERVINGS	CALORIES	MACROS
3	50	P: 2g C: 6g F: 3g

INGREDIENTS

3 Zucchini
1/2 tbsp Salt
1/2 tbsp Olive Oil

INSTRUCTIONS

***Also Needed: Parchment Paper

Preheat oven to 400F.

Slice zucchini into very thin slices (this depends on if your chips will crisp or not). Place zucchini in a bowl with olive oil. Add salt and then mix together.

Place zucchini slices on a cookie sheet without overlapping. Bake for approximately 2 hours, turning the pan halfway through.

Chicken and Broccoli Bowls

SERVINGS	CALORIES	MACROS
3	330	P: 53g C: 16g F: 7g

INGREDIENTS

3 cups Cauliflower Rice
3 1/2 cups Broccoli Florets
1 tbsp Grated Ginger
1/2 tsp Salt
1/2 tsp Garlic Powder
1/2 tsp Red Pepper Flakes
1/3 cup Coconut Aminos
1 pound Chicken Breast (Boneless, Skinless)

INSTRUCTIONS

In a large nonstick skillet, (once hot) add broccoli, ginger, salt, garlic powder, red pepper flakes and coconut aminos.

Cook over medium/high heat for 5 minutes until broccoli starts to soften.

Add the chicken and turn the heat to high.

Cook until chicken is fully cooked, stirring regularly, about 5 minutes.

Divide mixture evenly over cauliflower rice.

Thai Turkey Burger

SERVINGS	CALORIES	MACROS
3	240	P: 30g C: 5g F: 11g

INGREDIENTS

6 pieces Looseleaf Lettuce
1 pound 93% Ground Turkey
1/2 cup Carrots, Shredded
2 tbsp Chopped Cilantro
1 Green Onion
1/2 tsp Salt
1/2 tsp Garlic Powder
1/2 tsp Ground Ginger

INSTRUCTIONS

Chop green onion and cilantro.

Mix all ingredients in a medium bowl. Form into 3 patties.

In a hot nonstick pan, cook the burgers for approximately 5 minutes per side.

Wrap the burgers in looseleaf lettuce when ready to eat.

Meal Plan
TRADITIONAL/PALEO: 30P/50C/20F

1300 Calories	1500 Calories	1700 Calories
Daily Macros	**Daily Macros**	**Daily Macros**
Calories: 1305 Protein: 105g Carbs: 155g Fat: 28g	Calories: 1500 Protein: 113g Carbs: 180g Fat: 37g	Calories: 1721 Protein: 134g Carbs: 212g Fat: 40g
Breakfast	**Breakfast**	**Breakfast**
Spinach and Tomato Frittata	Spinach and Tomato Frittata 1 cup Raspberries	Spinach and Tomato Frittata 1 1/2 cup Raspberries
Snack	**Snack**	**Snack**
1 Banana 2 tbsp Almond Butter	1 Banana 2 tbsp Almond Butter	1 Banana 2 tbsp Almond Butter Protein Shake - 30 grams Protein Powder
Lunch	**Lunch**	**Lunch**
Buffalo Chicken Sweet Potatoes 1 cup Broccoli	Buffalo Chicken Sweet Potatoes 2 cups Broccoli	Buffalo Chicken Sweet Potatoes 2 cups Broccoli
Snack	**Snack**	**Snack**
1 1/4 cup Baby Carrots 1/3 cup Salsa	1 1/4 cup Baby Carrots 1/3 cup Salsa 1/2 oz Almonds	2 cup Baby Carrots 1/2 cup Salsa 1/2 oz Almonds
Dinner	**Dinner**	**Dinner**
Butternut Squash & Ground Turkey 6 oz Brussels Sprouts	Butternut Squash & Ground Turkey 8 oz Brussels Sprouts	Butternut Squash & Ground Turkey 8 oz Brussels Sprouts

Spinach and Tomato Frittata

SERVINGS	CALORIES	MACROS
3	160	P: 18g C: 7g F: 7g

INGREDIENTS

1 cup Egg Whites
4 Large Eggs
1/2 cup Plain Almond Milk, Unsweetened
2 cups Baby Spinach
1 cup Cherry Tomatoes
3 Garlic Cloves
1/2 tsp Onion Powder

INSTRUCTIONS

Preheat the oven to 375F.

Use a round, nonstick cooking dish.

Place the egg whites, eggs, almond milk, spinach, onion powder and minced garlic in a bowl and whisk together.

Pour the ingredients into the baking dish.

Slice the tomatoes and arrange the tomatoes in an even layer in the egg whites.

Bake for approximately 30 minutes or until the center is set.

Remove from the oven and cool in the pan 7-10 minutes.

Buffalo Chicken Sweet Potatoes

SERVINGS	CALORIES	MACROS
3	340	P: 36g C: 39g F: 4g

INGREDIENTS

3 Large Sweet Potatoes
2/3 pound Chicken Breast (Boneless, Skinless)
3/4 cup Buffalo Wing Sauce
1 tbsp Cornstarch

INSTRUCTIONS

Place the chicken in the bottom of the slow cooker.

Pour the hot sauce over the chicken.

Cover the slow cooker, then cook for 1 1/2 to 2 1/2 hours on high or 4 to 5 hours on low, until the chicken is cooked through.

Remove the chicken from crockpot and shred.

About 30 minutes before the chicken is done, bake the sweet potatoes: Preheat your oven to 400F.

Prick the sweet potatoes all over with a fork, then place them on a foil-lined baking sheet. Bake until the sweet potatoes are tender, about 45 minutes to 1 hour, depending upon the size of your sweet potato. Turn off the oven and leave the sweet potatoes inside to keep them warm.

Once the chicken is shredded and while the sweet potatoes bake, mix the cornstarch and 1 tablespoon water together to create a slurry. Add it to the cooking liquid in the slow cooker, then whisk to combine. Cover the slow cooker and cook on high for 30 minutes to allow the sauce to thicken, stirring once halfway through. Once thick, return the chicken to the slow cooker and toss to coat.

Divide the chicken evenly between the sweet potatoes.

Butternut Squash and Ground Turkey

SERVINGS	CALORIES	MACROS
3	280	P: 34g C: 26g F: 0g

INGREDIENTS

1 pound 99% Lean Ground Turkey
6 grams Garlic Clove
1/2 Onion
1 Red Bell Pepper
2 cups Butternut Squash
1 cup Diced Tomatoes
1 tsp Italian Seasoning

INSTRUCTIONS

In a nonstick skillet, add the turkey and cook, breaking up the meat, for 6-8 minutes.

Dice all the veggies.

Add the garlic, onion, and bell pepper. Cook for 4-5 minutes until onion begin to brown.

Add the butternut squash, tomatoes and Italian seasoning.

Cover the skillet and cook until the butternut squash is tender, about 6-8 minutes.

Add a touch of water if anything begins to burn.

Meal Plan
TRADITIONAL/PALEO: 45P/20C/35F

1300 Calories	1500 Calories	1700 Calories
Daily Macros	**Daily Macros**	**Daily Macros**
Calories: 1291 Protein: 142g Carbs: 67g Fat: 48g	Calories: 1502 Protein: 171g Carbs: 77g Fat: 55g	Calories: 1683 Protein: 188g Carbs: 92g Fat: 64g
Breakfast	**Breakfast**	**Breakfast**
Sweet Potato Toast	Sweet Potato Toast	Sweet Potato Toast
Snack	**Snack**	**Snack**
4 1/2 oz Tuna 2 Celery Stalks	4 1/2 oz Tuna 2 Celery Stalks Protein Shake - 30 grams Protein Powder	5 1/2 oz Tuna 6 Celery Stalks Protein Shake - 30 grams Protein Powder
Lunch	**Lunch**	**Lunch**
Lemon Baked Shrimp 6 oz Asparagus	Lemon Baked Shrimp 10 oz Asparagus	Lemon Baked Shrimp 12 oz Asparagus
Snack	**Snack**	**Snack**
1 Hard Boiled Egg 1 oz Almonds	2 Hard Boiled Eggs 1 oz Almonds	2 Hard Boiled Eggs 1 1/2 oz Almonds
Dinner	**Dinner**	**Dinner**
Hawaiian Chicken Burgers 1 cup Button Mushrooms	Hawaiian Chicken Burgers 1 cup Button Mushrooms	Hawaiian Chicken Burgers 1 1/2 cup Button Mushrooms

Sweet Potato Toast

SERVINGS	CALORIES	MACROS
1	340	P: 10g C: 32g F: 20g

INGREDIENTS

1 Large Egg
2 tbsp Avocado
4 oz Sweet Potato

INSTRUCTIONS

Place a slice of sweet potato in the toaster until tender.

While your "toast" is cooking, make one egg any style you wish.

Mash the avocado and spread on the sweet potato. Top with egg and add any spices you wish.

Lemon Baked Shrimp

SERVINGS	CALORIES	MACROS
3	170	P: 31g C: 2g F: 0g

INGREDIENTS

1 pound Shrimp (medium)
2 tbsp Fresh Italian Parsley
2 tbsp Fresh Lemon Juice
1 Garlic Raw Cloves
1 tsp Salt
1/4 tsp Ground Black Pepper

INSTRUCTIONS

***Also Needed: Parchment Paper

Preheat the oven to 400F and line a baking sheet with parchment paper.

Place onto the baking sheet. Top with lemon, garlic, salt, and pepper. Evenly coat the shrimp on both sides.

Bake in the preheated oven for 5 minutes. The shrimp should be pink.

Top with parsley and with additional lemon juice to taste if desired.

Hawaiian Chicken Burgers

SERVINGS	CALORIES	MACROS
3	280	P: 43g C: 10g F: 6g

INGREDIENTS

6 pieces Looseleaf Lettuce
1 pound Ground Chicken
1/2 cup Pineapple
2 tbsp Coconut Aminos
1/3 cup Green Onions, Chopped
3 tbsp Almond Flour

INSTRUCTIONS

In a large bowl, combine all the ingredients and form into 3 large burgers.

Then place into the freezer for at least 15 minutes.

In the meantime, preheat the grill to high heat.

Place the burger on nonstick grates.

Cook for 4-6 minutes per side.

If cooking on stovetop, use a nonstick skillet. Turn heat slightly above medium/high and place the burgers into the skillet, once hot.

Sear 2-3 minutes per side then transfer to the oven at 350 degrees for roughly 8-10 minutes until thoroughly cooked.

Wrap the burgers in looseleaf lettuce when ready to eat.

Meal Plan
FODMAP: 40P/40C/20F

1300 Calories	1500 Calories	1700 Calories
Daily Macros	**Daily Macros**	**Daily Macros**
Calories: 1296 Protein: 136g Carbs: 125g Fat: 28g	Calories: 1483 Protein: 153g Carbs: 149g Fat: 30g	Calories: 1695 Protein: 172g Carbs: 165g Fat: 38g
Breakfast	**Breakfast**	**Breakfast**
Turkey Breakfast Skillet	Turkey Breakfast Skillet 1 1/2 cups Raspberries	Turkey Breakfast Skillet 1 1/2 cups Raspberries
Snack	**Snack**	**Snack**
Tropical Orange Smoothie	Tropical Orange Smoothie	Tropical Orange Smoothie
Lunch	**Lunch**	**Lunch**
Beef Meatballs with Zoodles	Beef Meatballs with Zoodles	Beef Meatballs with Zoodles 2/3 cup Baby Carrots
Snack	**Snack**	**Snack**
2 oz Tuna 1 cup Cucumber	4 oz Tuna 1 1/2 cups Cucumber	6 oz Tuna 1 1/2 cups Cucumber 1/2 oz Almonds
Dinner	**Dinner**	**Dinner**
Slow Cooker Chicken Pot Pie	Slow Cooker Chicken Pot Pie	Slow Cooker Chicken Pot Pie

Turkey Breakfast Skillet

SERVINGS	CALORIES	MACROS
3	360	P: 32g C: 35g F: 11g

INGREDIENTS

1 cup Spinach
1/2 tsp Salt
1/4 tsp Ground Black Pepper
1/2 tsp Chili Powder
1 pound 93% Ground Turkey
2 cups Sweet Potato
1 Red Bell Pepper

INSTRUCTIONS

In a nonstick skillet, add diced sweet potato once hot. Cook for 5-7 minutes, stirring occasionally until they begin to brown but not cook through.

Add the ground turkey and salt and black pepper; brown turkey for about 5 minutes.

Dice bell pepper.

When turkey is cooked halfway through, add in bell pepper. Stir to combine and cook an additional 5-7 minutes.

Add in spinach and cook until wilted.

Taste and add any additional spices and seasonings as you wish.

Tropical Orange Smoothie

SERVINGS	CALORIES	MACROS
1	240	P: 3g C: 54g F: 1.5g

INGREDIENTS

1/2 cup Plain Almond Milk, Unsweetened
1/2 cup Frozen Pineapple
1 Unripe Banana
6 oz Fresh Orange

INSTRUCTIONS

Combine all ingredients into your blender. Blend on high until completely smooth.

Slow Cooker Chicken Stew

SERVINGS	CALORIES	MACROS
3	370	P: 51g C: 22g F: 9g

INGREDIENTS

4 oz Sweet Potato
2 cups Carrots
16 fl oz Chicken Stock
1/2 tsp Salt
1 Bay Leaf
1 pound Chicken Breast (Boneless, Skinless)
1/2 cup Lite Coconut Milk

INSTRUCTIONS

Dice carrots and sweet potato. Add all ingredients to slow cooker (except coconut milk) and mix.

Cook on high for 4-6 hours or low for 6-8 hours, or until the veggies are very tender and the chicken is cooked through.

Remove the chicken and cut into pieces. Add the chicken back to the slow cooker along with the coconut milk. Taste and add additional salt (or other spices) if desired. Let cook an additional 10-15 minutes.

Beef Meatballs with Zoodles

SERVINGS	CALORIES	MACROS
3	230	P: 34g C: 10g F: 6g

INGREDIENTS

1 pound 96% Extra Lean Ground Beef
1 tsp Coconut Aminos
1 tsp Balsamic Vinegar
1/2 tsp Dried Basil
1/2 tsp Dried Oregano
1 tbsp Coconut Flour
3 cups Grape Tomatoes
3 cups Zoodles (Zucchini Noodles)

INSTRUCTIONS

Preheat oven to 350F.

In a large bowl add all ingredients (except zucchini and tomatoes). Mix well and let sit for 5 minutes.

Form meat mixture into round balls. Brown all sides in a nonstick skillet.

After browning, place balls into oven-safe baking dish and cook for 10 minutes. Make sure meatballs are fully cooked.

While balls are cooking, add tomatoes to nonstick pan and cook until tomatoes start to deflate and are a little brown.

Finally, spiralize you zucchini or purchase already spiralized zoodles. (You can also grate your zucchini if that's more convenient).

Cook zoodles in a nonstick pan until soft, removing any excess water.

Assemble bowls together evenly with balls, tomatoes and zoodles.

Meal Plan
FODMAP: 30P/30C/40F

1300 Calories	1500 Calories	1700 Calories
Daily Macros	**Daily Macros**	**Daily Macros**
Calories: 1296 Protein: 101g Carbs: 92g Fat: 62g	Calories: 1506 Protein: 123g Carbs: 110g Fat: 68g	Calories: 1692 Protein: 126g Carbs: 130g Fat: 78g
Breakfast	**Breakfast**	**Breakfast**
Simple Raspberry Chia Pudding	Simple Raspberry Chia Pudding	Simple Raspberry Chia Pudding
Snack	**Snack**	**Snack**
1 cup Strawberries 1/2 cup Grapes	1 1/3 cups Strawberries 2/3 cup Grapes Protein Shake - 30 grams Protein Powder	1 1/3 cups Strawberries 1 cup Grapes Protein Shake - 30 grams Protein Powder
Lunch	**Lunch**	**Lunch**
Dijon Salmon 1 Zucchini	Dijon Salmon 1 Zucchini	Dijon Salmon 1 Zucchini 1/4 Avocado
Snack	**Snack**	**Snack**
2 cups Cherry Tomatoes 1/2 oz Almonds	2 cups Cherry Tomatoes 3/4 oz Almonds	2 cups Cherry Tomatoes 1 oz Almonds
Dinner	**Dinner**	**Dinner**
Simple Flank Steak 4 oz Sweet Potato	Simple Flank Steak 5 oz Sweet Potato	Simple Flank Steak 6 oz Sweet Potato

Simple Raspberry Chia Pudding

SERVINGS	CALORIES	MACROS
1	270	P: 11g C: 9g F: 18g

INGREDIENTS

3 tbsp Chia Seeds
1 cup Plain Almond Milk, Unsweetened
1/2 cup Frozen Raspberries

INSTRUCTIONS

Add all ingredients to a jar and shake. Place in the refrigerator overnight.

Dijon Salmon

SERVINGS	CALORIES	MACROS
3	300	P: 44g C: 0g F: 12g

INGREDIENTS

1 1/4 pounds Salmon
1/4 cup Fresh Italian Parsley
1/4 cup Dijon Mustard
1 tbsp Fresh Lemon Juice
1/2 tbsp Olive Oil

INSTRUCTIONS

***Also Needed: Parchment Paper

Preheat your oven to 375F.

Place the salmon on a parchment lined baking tray and set it aside.

Mix together the remaining ingredients in a small bowl and coat the top of the salmon evenly. Bake for approximately 20 minutes (depending on size and thickness).

Simple Flank Steak

SERVINGS	CALORIES	MACROS
3	350	P: 33g C: 6g F: 21g

INGREDIENTS

1 pound Beef, Flank Steak
1/3 cup Coconut Aminos
1/8 cup Olive Oil
2 tbsp Fresh Rosemary Leaf
1 tbsp Balsamic Vinegar

INSTRUCTIONS

***NOTE: Meat needs to marinate overnight
****Also Needed: Ziploc Bag

Whisk all ingredients together in a bowl (except steak).

Place steak in a plastic bag and pour marinade in. Squeeze out excess air and tightly seal bag. Place in refrigerator and let marinade overnight.

When you're ready to cook the steak remove it from the marinade.

Add the meat to a nonstick skillet and cook until reached desired doneness.

Place aside and let the steak rest for about 10 minutes. Then, slice the steak against the grain.

Meal Plan
VEGETARIAN: 50P/30C/20F

1300 Calories	1500 Calories	1700 Calories

Daily Macros

Calories: 1334
Protein: 164g
Carbs: 101g
Fat: 32g

Breakfast

Microwave Egg White Omelet
2/3 cup Nonfat Cottage Cheese

Snack

1 cup Nonfat Greek Yogurt
30 grams Protein Powder
1/4 cup Blueberries

Lunch

Balsamic Tofu
1 cup Broccoli

Snack

Protein Shake -
30 grams Protein Powder
1/4 cup Edamame

Dinner

Mango Tempeh Lettuce Wraps

Daily Macros

Calories: 1498
Protein: 182g
Carbs: 120g
Fat: 35g

Breakfast

Microwave Egg White Omelet
1 cup Nonfat Cottage Cheese

Snack

1 cup Nonfat Greek Yogurt
30 grams Protein Powder
1/4 cup Blueberries

Lunch

Balsamic Tofu
1 cup Broccoli

Snack

Protein Shake -
30 grams Protein Powder
1/2 cup Edamame

Dinner

Mango Tempeh Lettuce Wraps
4 oz Green Beans

Daily Macros

Calories: 1720
Protein: 206g
Carbs: 129g
Fat: 44g

Breakfast

Microwave Egg White Omelet
1 cup Nonfat Cottage Cheese

Snack

1 1/3 cup Nonfat Greek Yogurt
30 grams Protein Powder
1/4 cup Blueberries
1 Hard Boiled Egg

Lunch

Balsamic Tofu
1 cup Broccoli

Snack

Protein Shake -
30 grams Protein Powder
2/3 cup Edamame
1 Mozzarella Cheese Stick

Dinner

Mango Tempeh Lettuce Wraps
4 oz Green Beans

Microwave Egg White Omelet

SERVINGS	CALORIES	MACROS
1	140	P: 22g C: 2g F: 3g

INGREDIENTS

2 tbsp Reduced Fat Mozzarella Cheese, Shredded
2/3 cup Egg Whites
1 tbsp Skim Milk
1/4 cup Spinach
2 tbsp Bell Pepper
2 tbsp Broccoli Florets

INSTRUCTIONS

In a microwave safe mug, whisk together egg whites and milk. Chop veggies and add the remaining ingredients to the mug. Microwave for about 1 minute 30 seconds or until done.

Balsamic Tofu

SERVINGS	CALORIES	MACROS
3	260	P: 22g C: 16g F: 13g

INGREDIENTS

24 oz Firm Tofu
1/2 cups Balsamic Vinegar
2 tablespoons Coconut Aminos (coconut Secret)
1/2 tablespoons Raw Local Honey
1/2 tablespoons Olive Oil 1 Tbsp
1 serving Garlic Raw Cloves (3)

INSTRUCTIONS

Mix all ingredients in a bowl besides tofu. After pressing the water out of the tofu, slice up the block and add to the marinade.

Preheat a skillet to medium-high heat and add in the marinade.

Bring it to a boil then simmer for about 10 minutes until it starts to thicken.

Then place the tofu on the pan and cook about 3-4 minutes per side.

Mango Tempeh Lettuce Wraps

SERVINGS	CALORIES	MACROS
3	330	P: 30g C: 33g F: 10g

INGREDIENTS

16 oz Lightlife Tempeh
2 tablespoons Hoisin Sauce
1 tablespoons Lime Juice
1/3 cups Mango, Raw
1/2 cups Cucumber - Sliced/diced
1/2 oz Cashews
6 leaf Lettuce, Looseleaf, Raw

INSTRUCTIONS

****NOTE: Each serving is 2 lettuce Wraps

In a nonstick skillet, add the tempeh and cook, stirring often, until lightly browned, about 3 minutes.

Stir in the hoisin sauce and lime juice; remove from heat.

Chop the mango, cucumber and cashews.

Divide the tempeh, mango, cucumber and cashews into lettuce leaves.

Meal Plan
VEGETARIAN: 35P/45C/20F

1300 Calories	1500 Calories	1700 Calories

Daily Macros

Calories: 1320
Protein: 115g
Carbs: 151g
Fat: 31g

Breakfast

Strawberry Protein Smoothie

Snack

1 Hard Boiled Egg
1 Cheddar Cheese Stick

Lunch

Quinoa Stuffed Bell Peppers
1/2 cup Nonfat Cottage Cheese

Snack

Protein Shake -
30 grams Protein Powder
1 cup Raspberries

Dinner

Tempeh Acorn Squash
4 oz Green Beans

Daily Macros

Calories: 1511
Protein: 130g
Carbs: 171g
Fat: 36g

Breakfast

Strawberry Protein Smoothie

Snack

2 Hard Boiled Eggs
1 Cheddar Cheese Stick

Lunch

Quinoa Stuffed Bell Peppers
3/4 cup Nonfat Cottage Cheese

Snack

Protein Shake -
30 grams Protein Powder
1 1/2 cups Raspberries

Dinner

Tempeh Acorn Squash
8 oz Green Beans

Daily Macros

Calories: 1724
Protein: 151g
Carbs: 204g
Fat: 36g

Breakfast

Strawberry Protein Smoothie
1/2 cup Nonfat Greek Yogurt
1/4 cup Blueberries

Snack

2 Hard Boiled Eggs
1 Cheddar Cheese Stick

Lunch

Quinoa Stuffed Bell Peppers
1 cup Nonfat Cottage Cheese

Snack

Protein Shake -
30 grams Protein Powder
1 1/2 cups Raspberries
1 cup Baby Carrots

Dinner

Tempeh Acorn Squash
8 oz Green Beans

Strawberry Protein Smoothie

SERVINGS	CALORIES	MACROS
1	360	P: 27g C: 50g F: 6g

INGREDIENTS

30 grams Vega Protein And Greens, Vanilla
1 cup Strawberries
1/2 cup Old Fashioned Oats
1 tsp Agave
1 cup Plain Almond Milk, Unsweetened

INSTRUCTIONS

Add all ingredients to a blender and blend until smooth. Add ice cubes for a thicker consistency.

Tempeh Acorn Squash

SERVINGS	CALORIES	MACROS
3	330	P: 31g C: 38g F: 8g

INGREDIENTS

1 Acorn Squash
16 oz Tempeh
3 grams Garlic Clove
3 tbsp Tomato Paste
4 tbsp Tomato Sauce
1 tsp Coconut Aminos

INSTRUCTIONS

Preheat oven to 375F.

Cut acorn squash and sprinkle with salt and pepper. Place cut side down on a baking sheet, and bake for 20-30 minutes, or until tender.

While the squash is baking, heat a medium saucepan over medium heat. Add garlic, and cook for 30 seconds until fragrant.

Add finely chopped tempeh, and saute 2 minutes. Add tomato paste, tomato sauce, and coconut aminos to combine. Remove from heat.

Once squash is cooked, cut into cubes and divide evenly with tempeh.

Quinoa Stuffed Bell Peppers

SERVINGS	CALORIES	MACROS
3	170	P: 8g C: 28g F: 2g

INGREDIENTS

1 cup Cooked Quinoa
1/2 cup Chickpeas
1 Zucchini
1/2 cup Button Mushrooms
1/2 tsp Cumin
1/2 tsp Garlic Powder
1/2 tsp Onion Powder
3 Red Bell Pepper

INSTRUCTIONS

****Also Needed: Parchment Paper

Preheat oven to 400F. Line a baking tray with parchment paper.

Chop all vegetables.

In a large bowl, combine cooked quinoa, chickpeas, zucchini, mushrooms, cumin, garlic powder, onion powder, salt and pepper to taste.

Hollow out the bell peppers and cut in half.

Spoon the filling into each half of the bell peppers.

Place on prepared baking dish and bake until the peppers are tender and the filling is heated through, about 30 minutes or longer if you prefer the red bell peppers to be softer.

Meal Plan
VEGETARIAN: 45P/35C/20F

1300 Calories	1500 Calories	1700 Calories

Daily Macros

Calories: 1290
Protein: 149g
Carbs: 119g
Fat: 32g

Breakfast

Egg White & Veggie Burrito
1/2 cup Cherry Tomatoes

Snack

Protein Shake -
30 grams Protein Powder
1 Hard Boiled Egg

Lunch

Tempeh BLT Wrap

Snack

Protein Shake -
30 grams Protein Powder
1 cup Strawberries
3/4 cup Nonfat Cottage Cheese

Dinner

Sesame Garlic Tofu
1/2 cup Cauliflower Rice
7 oz Fresh Asparagus

Daily Macros

Calories: 1490
Protein: 173g
Carbs: 143g
Fat: 33g

Breakfast

Egg White & Veggie Burrito
1/2 cup Cherry Tomatoes

Snack

Protein Shake -
30 grams Protein Powder
1 Hard Boiled Egg
2/3 cup Nonfat Greek Yogurt
1 cup Raspberries

Lunch

Tempeh BLT Wrap

Snack

Protein Shake -
30 grams Protein Powder
1 cup Strawberries
1 cup Nonfat Cottage Cheese

Dinner

Sesame Garlic Tofu
1/2 cup Cauliflower Rice
7 oz Fresh Asparagus

Daily Macros

Calories: 1691
Protein: 193g
Carbs: 158g
Fat: 41g

Breakfast

Egg White & Veggie Burrito
1/2 cup Cherry Tomatoes
1/2 oz Almonds

Snack

Protein Shake -
30 grams Protein Powder
1 Hard Boiled Egg
1 cup Nonfat Greek Yogurt
1 cup Raspberries

Lunch

Tempeh BLT Wrap
1 Zucchini

Snack

Protein Shake -
30 grams Protein Powder
1 cup Strawberries
1 1/4 cup Nonfat Cottage Cheese

Dinner

Sesame Garlic Tofu
1/2 cup Cauliflower Rice
7 oz Fresh Asparagus

Egg White & Veggie Burritos

SERVINGS	CALORIES	MACROS
3	200	P: 23g C: 15g F: 3g

INGREDIENTS

3 Mission Carb Balance Flour Tortillas
4 oz Button Mushrooms
1/2 Red Bell Pepper
1/8 cup Diced Onion
1/2 tbsp Minced Garlic
1 cup Baby Spinach
1 1/2 oz Reduced-Fat Mozzarella Cheese, Shredded
16 oz Egg Whites

INSTRUCTIONS

In a large nonstick skillet, saute mushrooms, bell pepper, onion, and garlic until tender (about 5 minutes).

Add in spinach and cook until wilted. Remove veggies and set aside.

In the same pan, add your egg whites and scramble until fully cooked.

Divide your egg whites and veggies evenly between tortillas. Top with cheese and wrap.

Tempeh BLT Wrap

SERVINGS	CALORIES	MACROS
3	270	P: 29g C: 23g F: 8g

INGREDIENTS

6 pieces Looseleaf Lettuce
16 oz Tempeh
1 1/2 tbsp Coconut Aminos
1 1/2 tsp Agave
1/2 tsp Onion Powder
1/8 tsp Cumin
1/3 cup Tomato

INSTRUCTIONS

Whisk together coconut aminos, agave, cumin, onion powder, and a pinch of black pepper into a medium bowl.

Add tempeh slices and marinade for approximately 15 minutes.

In a large non-stick pan over medium heat, add tempeh slices and sear each side for 3-4 minutes on each side until slightly blackened at the edges.

Assemble lettuce wraps evenly with tempeh and diced tomato. You can add mustard if you'd like.

Sesame Garlic Tofu

SERVINGS	CALORIES	MACROS
3	250	P: 19g C: 25g F: 9g

INGREDIENTS

21 oz Firm Tofu
3 tbsp Cornstarch
1/3 cup Coconut Aminos
3 tbsp Water
3 tsp Honey
2 1/2 tsp Chili Garlic Sauce
3/4 tbsp Rice Wine Vinegar
3 tsp Cornstarch

INSTRUCTIONS

Drain the tofu of excess water. After drained completely, slice into cubes and add to a large bowl. Sprinkle with the 3 tbsp of cornstarch and mix completely.

In a large, nonstick skillet add tofu cubes and brown on all sides.

While tofu is cooking, whisk together the ingredients for the sauce.

Once the tofu has browned and crisped up on all sides, add the sauce to the skillet and it should start to thicken immediately.

Toss the tofu around to coat then remove from heat.

Meal Plan
VEGAN: 45P/30C/25F

1300 Calories	1500 Calories	1700 Calories
Daily Macros	**Daily Macros**	**Daily Macros**
Calories: 1284 Protein: 143g Carbs: 104g Fat: 38g	Calories: 1491 Protein: 166g Carbs: 121g Fat: 44g	Calories: 1693 Protein: 187g Carbs: 138g Fat: 50g
Breakfast	**Breakfast**	**Breakfast**
Chickpea Omelet 2/3 cup Edamame	Chickpea Omelet 2/3 cup Edamame	Chickpea Omelet 2/3 cup Edamame
Snack	**Snack**	**Snack**
Protein Shake - 30 grams Protein Powder 1 cup Strawberries	Protein Shake - 30 grams Protein Powder 1 cup Strawberries Baked Tempeh Chips	Protein Shake - 30 grams Protein Powder 2 servings Baked Tempeh Chips
Lunch	**Lunch**	**Lunch**
Blackened Tofu 6 oz Asparagus 1 cup Cauliflower Rice	Blackened Tofu 7 oz Asparagus 1 cup Cauliflower Rice	Blackened Tofu 7 oz Asparagus 1 cup Cauliflower Rice
Snack	**Snack**	**Snack**
Protein Shake - 30 grams Protein Powder 1 oz Almonds	Protein Shake - 30 grams Protein Powder 1 oz Almonds	Protein Shake - 30 grams Protein Powder 1 oz Almonds
Dinner	**Dinner**	**Dinner**
Peppers & Onions Seitan	Peppers & Onions Seitan	Peppers & Onions Seitan 1 cup Strawberries

Chickpea Omelet

SERVINGS	CALORIES	MACROS
1	140	P: 10g C: 21g F: 2.5g

INGREDIENTS

1 tbsp Nutritional Yeast
1/4 cup Chickpea Flour
1/3 cup Water
1/4 tsp Salt
1/2 cup Spinach
1/8 cup Button Mushrooms
1/8 cup Broccoli Florets

INSTRUCTIONS

Mix chickpea flour, nutritional yeast, salt and water and stir until there are no lumps.

Dice up veggies.

In a nonstick pan, saute the veggies on medium-low for about 3-5 minutes until they become tender.

Remove the veggies and add them to the batter; mix well.

Turn up the heat to medium and pour the batter in the skillet like you would a large pancake and cook for about 5 minutes until the top of the omelet no longer looks wet.

Carefully loosen up the omelet with a spatula and flip the omelet to the other side and cook for 3-5 more minutes until it is no longer soft in the middle.

Make sure the omelet is fully cooked.

Baked Tempeh Chips

SERVINGS	CALORIES	MACROS
3	200	P: 22g C: 16g F: 6g

INGREDIENTS

12 oz Tempeh
1 tsp Onion Powder
1 tsp Garlic Powder
1 tsp Paprika
1/4 tsp Salt
2 tsp Coconut Sugar

INSTRUCTIONS

Preheat oven to 375F.

Combine onion powder, garlic powder, paprika, salt and coconut sugar in a small bowl.

Cut tempeh into even triangles.

Place tempeh slices on a nonstick baking sheet. Sprinkle half of the spice blend over the tempeh. Flip tempeh and sprinkle on the remaining spice blend.

Bake for 10 minutes. Flip and bake for another 7-10 minutes or until tempeh is golden brown and crisp.

Be sure to watch closely in the final few minutes because the tempeh can quickly go from golden brown to burnt.

Blackened Tofu

SERVINGS	CALORIES	MACROS
3	150	P: 14g C: 5g F: 7g

INGREDIENTS

16 oz Firm Tofu
2 tsp Dijon Mustard
2 tsp Paprika
1/2 tsp Cayenne Pepper
1/2 tsp Cumin
1/2 tsp Dried Thyme

INSTRUCTIONS

Press the excess liquid from the tofu.

Preheat oven to 375F.

Cut tofu into cubes and place in a medium bowl and add dijon mustard. Mix well. Then, add all spices and mix well again.

Bake on a nonstick baking sheet for 20-25 minutes flipping halfway through.

Peppers & Onions Seitan

SERVINGS	CALORIES	MACROS
3	290	P: 48g C: 20g F: 3g

INGREDIENTS

1 Onion
2 Red Bell Pepper
20 oz Seitan
1 tbsp Ketchup
1 tbsp Coconut Aminos
1/2 tsp Cumin
1/2 tsp Garlic Powder
1 tsp Rice Wine Vinegar

INSTRUCTIONS

Dice the bell pepper and onions.

In a nonstick skillet, add the diced onion, cook for a few minutes until it begins to soften.

Add the bell pepper to the skillet and cook for another 5 minutes.

While the onions and pepper cook, make the sauce in a small bowl.

Combine the ketchup, coconut aminos, cumin, garlic powder and vinegar. Whisk together and set aside.

After the bell pepper has cooked for 5 minutes, add the seitan to the skillet.

Add the sauce, and stir so that the seitan, onions and peppers are well combined.

Cook the seitan for 5 minutes, stirring occasionally, then the dish is ready to serve.

Meal Plan
VEGAN: 30P/35C/35F

1300 Calories	1500 Calories	1700 Calories
Daily Macros	**Daily Macros**	**Daily Macros**
Calories: 1326	Calories: 1495	Calories: 1691
Protein: 108g	Protein: 116g	Protein: 125g
Carbs: 122g	Carbs: 135g	Carbs: 153g
Fat: 48g	Fat: 58g	Fat: 67g
Breakfast	**Breakfast**	**Breakfast**
Tofu Scramble	Tofu Scramble	Tofu Scramble
Snack	**Snack**	**Snack**
Protein Shake -	Protein Shake -	Protein Shake -
30 grams Protein Powder	30 grams Protein Powder	30 grams Protein Powder
1/2 cup Edamame	2/3 cup Edamame	2/3 cup Edamame
Lunch	**Lunch**	**Lunch**
Cucumber Hummus Wrap	Cucumber Hummus Wrap	Cucumber Hummus Wrap
	1/4 Avocado	1/4 Avocado
Snack	**Snack**	**Snack**
2/3 oz Almonds	1 oz Almonds	1 oz Almonds
6 Cherry Tomatoes	12 Cherry Tomatoes	12 Cherry Tomatoes
Dinner	**Dinner**	**Dinner**
Balsamic Tempeh & Veggies	Balsamic Tempeh & Veggies	Balsamic Tempeh & Veggies
1/3 cup Cooked Quinoa	1/3 cup Cooked Quinoa	1/3 cup Cooked Quinoa

Tofu Scramble

SERVINGS	CALORIES	MACROS
3	190	P: 19g C: 10g F: 9g

INGREDIENTS

20 oz Firm Tofu
1/2 cup Diced Onion
1/2 cup Bell Pepper (Red and Green)
1/2 cup Button Mushrooms
2 tsp Ground Turmeric
1 tsp Coconut Aminos
1 tsp Nutritional Yeast
1/2 cup Spinach

INSTRUCTIONS

Drain liquid from tofu. Once drained, crumble tofu into a bowl and set aside.

Dice mushrooms, onions, and bell pepper.

In a nonstick pan, saute onion, bell pepper, and mushrooms for approximately 3-4 minutes.

Add crumbed tofu to pan with veggies.

Add turmeric, nutritional yeast and coconut aminos. Sauté for about 3 minutes.

Add baby spinach, cover pan with lid, and allow leaves to wilt, approximately 2 minutes.

Cucumber Hummus Wrap

SERVINGS	CALORIES	MACROS
2	300	P: 16g C: 40g F: 9g

INGREDIENTS

1/4 cup Cucumber
1 cup Arugula
1 1/2 cup Chickpeas
2 tsp Tahini
1/2 Lemon, Juice
1/2 tsp Chili Powder
3 grams Garlic
1/4 cup Water
2 Mission Carb Balance Flour Tortillas

INSTRUCTIONS

Rinse and drain chickpeas. Put hummus ingredients in a blender (garlic, chili powder, lemon juice, tahini, chickpeas). Add water gradually, blend until smooth.

Add hummus to the middle of a tortilla and top with arugula and chopped cucumber.

Balsamic Tempeh & Veggies

SERVINGS	CALORIES	MACROS
3	370	P: 32g C: 33g F: 13g

INGREDIENTS

3 tbsp Balsamic Vinegar
1 tbsp Olive Oil
1 tbsp Italian Seasoning
8 oz Button Mushrooms
2 Zucchini
2 Carrots
2 Red Bell Pepper
16 oz Tempeh

INSTRUCTIONS

***Also Needed: Parchment Paper

Preheat oven to 425F. Line a baking sheet with parchment and set aside.

Whisk together the vinegar, oil and spices.

Add the chopped vegetables and tempeh to a large mixing bowl, then pour dressing over top. Mix well.

Transfer everything to the baking sheet and roast for 25 - 30 minutes until the vegetables are tender and the tempeh has started to brown.

Meal Plan
VEGAN: 25P/55C/20F

1300 Calories	1500 Calories	1700 Calories
Daily Macros	**Daily Macros**	**Daily Macros**
Calories: 1326 Protein: 89g Carbs: 180g Fat: 34g	Calories: 1506 Protein: 97g Carbs: 206g Fat: 38g	Calories: 1694 Protein: 107g Carbs: 233g Fat: 42g
Breakfast	**Breakfast**	**Breakfast**
Vegan Breakfast Hash	Vegan Breakfast Hash	Vegan Breakfast Hash
Snack	**Snack**	**Snack**
Protein Shake - 30 grams Protein Powder	Protein Shake - 30 grams Protein Powder 1 cup Raspberries	Protein Shake - 30 grams Protein Powder 1 1/2 cups Raspberries
Lunch	**Lunch**	**Lunch**
Sticky Tofu Bowls	Sticky Tofu Bowls 1/2 cup Broccoli	Sticky Tofu Bowls 1 1/2 cups Broccoli
Snack	**Snack**	**Snack**
1/3 oz Almonds 1/2 cup Edamame	1/2 oz Almonds 2/3 cup Edamame	1/2 oz Almonds 1 cup Edamame
Dinner	**Dinner**	**Dinner**
Lentil Chili	Lentil Chili	Lentil Chili

Vegan Breakfast Hash

SERVINGS	CALORIES	MACROS
3	340	P: 12g C: 57g F: 8g

INGREDIENTS

1 pound Sweet Potato
1/2 Onion
1 1/2 cups Bell Pepper (Red, Green)
15 oz Chickpeas
1 tbsp Olive Oil
1 tsp Garlic Powder

INSTRUCTIONS

***Also Needed: Parchment Paper

Preheat oven to 425F. Line a sheet pan with parchment paper.

Place the diced sweet potatoes, onion, bell peppers and chickpeas on the center of the sheet pan, drizzle with olive oil, garlic powder, a pinch of salt and pepper, toss well to coat. Arrange the sweet potato mixture in a single layer.

Place sheet pan in the oven, on the center rack, and cook for 20 minutes, mixing halfway through.

Turn heat up to 500F, stir a second time and continue baking for another 20 minutes, mixing halfway through.

Sticky Tofu Bowl

SERVINGS	CALORIES	MACROS
3	260	P: 17g C: 26g F: 13g

INGREDIENTS

2 cups Cherry Tomatoes
1/2 Avocado
1 cup Cucumber
1/4 cup Carrots, Shredded
1 cup Green and Red Cabbage
16 oz Firm Tofu
1 tbsp Coconut Aminos
2 tbsp Hoisin Sauce
1 tsp Sriracha

INSTRUCTIONS

Drain all liquid from tofu.

Chop the tofu into cubes, and place in a nonstick, hot pan on medium-high heat.

Allow to brown, approximately 3-5 minutes, and then flip the cubes to brown on each side.

Once each side is golden brown and crispy, turn off the heat, and toss with coconut aminos, hoisin sauce and Sriracha.

Chop all veggies and slice avocado.

In separate containers divide everything evenly: cabbage, carrots, cucumber, cherry tomatoes and tofu.

Lentil Chili

SERVINGS	CALORIES	MACROS
3	410	P: 25g C: 76g F: 1g

INGREDIENTS

1/2 cup Corn
1/2 cup Black Beans
1 cup Diced Onion
1 Red Bell Pepper
1 Garlic Cloves
2 tsp Chili Powder
8 oz Black Lentils, Uncooked
14 1/2 oz Diced Tomatoes
32 oz Vegetable Cooking Stock

INSTRUCTIONS

Add all ingredients to a large pot, mix well and bring to a boil.

Turn the heat to medium-low and simmer for 30 minutes (leaving partially covered) or until lentils are tender.

MACRO {HACKS}

CHARTS AND RESOURCES

Macro Cheat Sheet

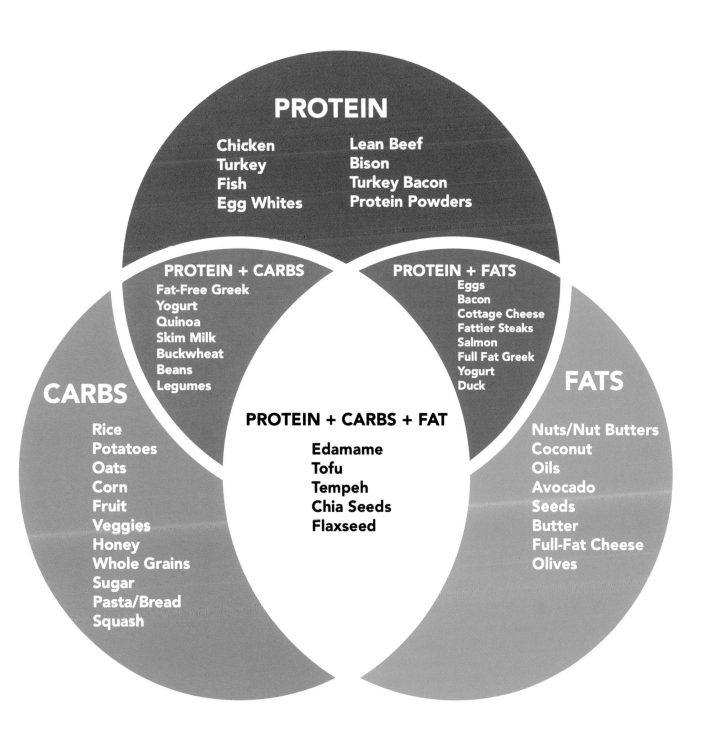

PROTEIN
Chicken
Turkey
Fish
Egg Whites
Lean Beef
Bison
Turkey Bacon
Protein Powders

PROTEIN + CARBS
Fat-Free Greek
Yogurt
Quinoa
Skim Milk
Buckwheat
Beans
Legumes

PROTEIN + FATS
Eggs
Bacon
Cottage Cheese
Fattier Steaks
Salmon
Full Fat Greek
Yogurt
Duck

CARBS
Rice
Potatoes
Oats
Corn
Fruit
Veggies
Honey
Whole Grains
Sugar
Pasta/Bread
Squash

PROTEIN + CARBS + FAT
Edamame
Tofu
Tempeh
Chia Seeds
Flaxseed

FATS
Nuts/Nut Butters
Coconut
Oils
Avocado
Seeds
Butter
Full-Fat Cheese
Olives

Complementary Proteins

Many plant sources provide incomplete amino acid chains, but when combined, can create complete proteins. We call these combinations complementary proteins!

LYSINE- This amino acid aids in calcium absorption and plays a major role in building muscle protein. It also aids in recovery and helps your body produce hormones, enzymes and antibodies.

THREONINE- This amino acid plays an important part in the function of many proteins, such as tooth enamel, collagen and elastin. It is also important for our nervous system as well as useful to help with intestinal disorders and indigestion.

METHIONINE- This amino acid is required for growth and tissue repair. A sulphur-containing amino acid, it improves the tone and pliability of our skin and hair while strengthening our nails. It is also involved in may detoxifying processes and can help prevent excess fat buildup in the liver.

OTHER- There are 6 other essential amino acids, histidine, isoleucine, leucine, phenylalanine, tryptophan, that are required to create a complete protein. Plant-sources are not commonly as deficit in these as Lysine, Threonine and Methionine.

These are some great ways to combine the incomplete proteins to the right into complementary proteins!

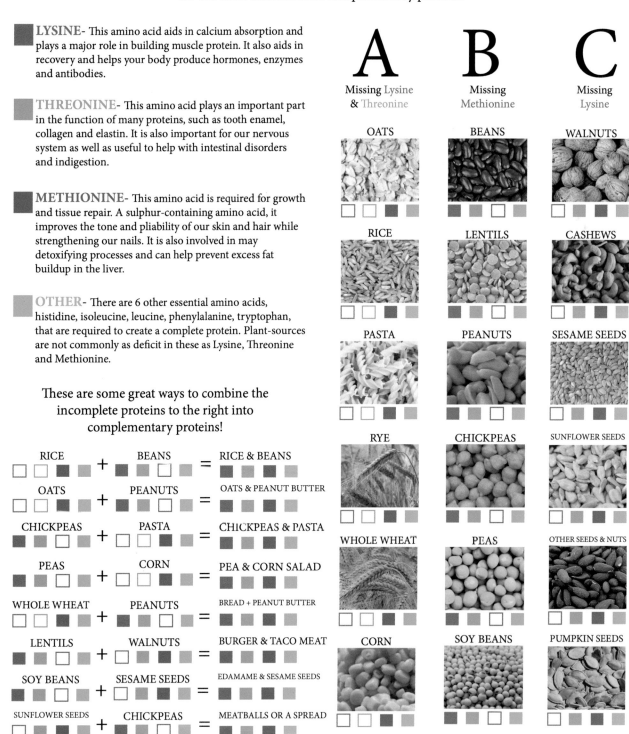

RICE + BEANS = RICE & BEANS

OATS + PEANUTS = OATS & PEANUT BUTTER

CHICKPEAS + PASTA = CHICKPEAS & PASTA

PEAS + CORN = PEA & CORN SALAD

WHOLE WHEAT + PEANUTS = BREAD + PEANUT BUTTER

LENTILS + WALNUTS = BURGER & TACO MEAT

SOY BEANS + SESAME SEEDS = EDAMAME & SESAME SEEDS

SUNFLOWER SEEDS + CHICKPEAS = MEATBALLS OR A SPREAD

PUMPKIN SEEDS + PEANUTS = TRAIL MIX

A Missing Lysine & Threonine

B Missing Methionine

C Missing Lysine

OATS — RICE — PASTA — RYE — WHOLE WHEAT — CORN

BEANS — LENTILS — PEANUTS — CHICKPEAS — PEAS — SOY BEANS

WALNUTS — CASHEWS — SESAME SEEDS — SUNFLOWER SEEDS — OTHER SEEDS & NUTS — PUMPKIN SEEDS

184

Know Your Veggie Protein

(Based On 1 Serving)

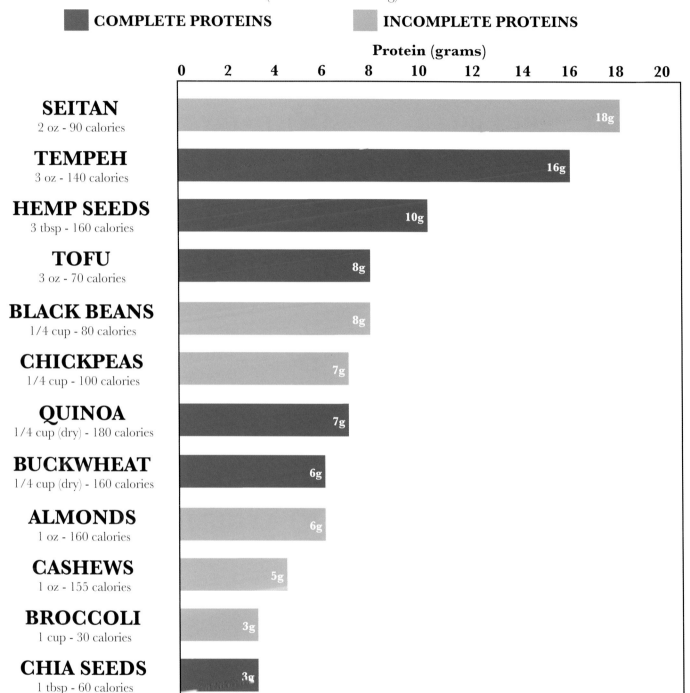

COMPLETE PROTEINS   **INCOMPLETE PROTEINS**

Protein (grams)

| | | | | | | | | | | |
| 0 | 2 | 4 | 6 | 8 | 10 | 12 | 14 | 16 | 18 | 20 |

SEITAN
2 oz - 90 calories — 18g

TEMPEH
3 oz - 140 calories — 16g

HEMP SEEDS
3 tbsp - 160 calories — 10g

TOFU
3 oz - 70 calories — 8g

BLACK BEANS
1/4 cup - 80 calories — 8g

CHICKPEAS
1/4 cup - 100 calories — 7g

QUINOA
1/4 cup (dry) - 180 calories — 7g

BUCKWHEAT
1/4 cup (dry) - 160 calories — 6g

ALMONDS
1 oz - 160 calories — 6g

CASHEWS
1 oz - 155 calories — 5g

BROCCOLI
1 cup - 30 calories — 3g

CHIA SEEDS
1 tbsp - 60 calories — 3g

PALEO DIET 101

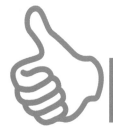
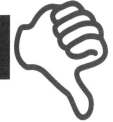

EAT THIS!	AVOID THIS!

 ## VEGETABLES
Sweet Potatoes, Yams, Acorn Squash, Butternut Squash, Beets, Kale, Bok Choy, Arugula, Spinach, Celery, Asparagus, Mushrooms, Cucumbers, Cauliflower, Broccoli, Zucchini, Cabbage, Brussel Sprouts, Carrots, Artichoke, Pumpkin

 ## FRUITS
Mangos, Apples, Bananas, Grapes, Peaches, Oranges, Pineapple, Pears, Tangerines, Dates, Strawberries, Watermelon, Raspberries, Kiwi, Blackberries, Plums, Blueberries, Lemon, Lime

 ## MEATS & SEAFOOD
Beef, Steak, Bison, Pork, Lamb, Chicken, Turkey, Tuna, Salmon, Cod, Tilapia, Shrimp

 ## EGG, NUTS, SEEDS
Almonds, Cashews, Pistachios, Walnuts, Pecans, Macadamia Nuts, Pumpkin Seeds, Sunflower Seeds, Flax Seeds, Chia Seeds

 ## DAIRY
Milk, Cheese, Yogurt, Butter, Ice Cream

 ## Processed Sugar
Artificial and Refined Sweeteners

 ## GRAINS
Quinoa, Bread, Pasta, Rice, Corn, Wheat, Oats, Buckwheat

 ## Vegetable & Seed Oils
Corn Oil, Vegetable Oil, Canola Oil, Margarine, Peanut Oil, Cotton Seed Oil

 ## PROCESSED FOODS
Bacon, Deli Meat, Chips, Pizza, Packaged Foods

 ## LEGUMES
Beans, Peanuts, Lentils, Soy

FODMAP Food List

Low FODMAP Foods

VEGETABLES	FRUITS	DAIRY & ALTERNATIVES	PROTEIN	BREADS/CEREAL PRODUCTS	SUGARS/ SWEETENERS	NUTS/SEEDS
Alfalfa Sprouts	Oranges	Brie	Beef	Rice	Dark Chocolate	Almonds
Bean Sprouts	Grapes	Camembert	Pork	Rice Bran	Maple Syrup	Macadamia
Bell Pepper	Honeydew	Feta Cheese	Chicken	Oats	Rice Melt Syrup	Peanuts
Carrot	Cantaloupe	Almond Milk	Fish	Oat Bran	Table Sugar	Pine Nuts
Green Beans	Banana	Rice Milk	Eggs	Quinoa		Walnuts
Bok Choy	Blueberries	Coconut Milk	Tofu	Corn Flour		Pumpkin Seeds
Cucumber	Grapefruit		Tempeh	Sourdough Spelt Bread		
Lettuce	Kiwi			Gluten-Free Bread & Pasta		
Tomato	Lemon					
Zucchini	Lime					
Bamboo Shoots	Strawberries					
Eggplant	Unripe Banana					
Ginger						
Chives						
Olives						
Parsnips						
Potatoes						
Turnips						

High FODMAP Foods

VEGETABLES	FRUITS	DAIRY & ALTERNATIVES	PROTEIN	BREADS/CEREAL PRODUCTS	SUGARS/ SWEETENERS	NUTS/SEEDS
Onions	Peaches	Milk	Chorizo	Wheat and Rye:	High Fructose	Cashews
Garlic	Apricots	Soft Cheese	Sausage	Breads	Corn Syrup	Pistachios
Cabbage	Nectarines	Yogurt	Some Processed	Cereals	Honey	
Broccoli	Plums	Ice cream	Meats	Pastas	Agave Nectar	
Cauliflower	Prunes	Custard		Crackers	Sorbitol	
Snow Peas	Mangoes	Pudding		Pizza	Xylitol	
Asparagus	Apples	Cottage Cheese			Maltitol	
Artichokes	Pears				Mannitol	
Leeks	Watermelon				Isomalt	
Beans	Cherries					
Celery	Blackberries					
Sweet Corn	Ripe Banana					
Brussels Sprouts						
Mushrooms						

A Guide To Portion Sizes

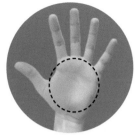

PALM = Approximately 3 ounces
Poultry, Meat, Fish

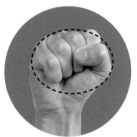

FIST = Approximately 1 cup
Rice, Pasta, Fruit, Veggies

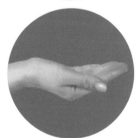

CUPPED HAND = Approximately 1/2 cup
Beans, Potatoes

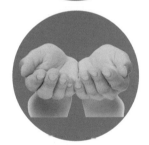

2 CUPPED HANDS = Approximately 1 Ounce
Chips, Popcorn, Pretzels

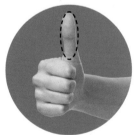

THUMB = Approximately 1 Ounce or 1 Tbsp
Peanut Butter, Hard Cheese

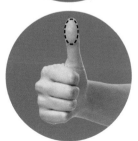

THUMB TIP = Approximately 1 Teaspoon
Cooking Oil, Mayo, Butter